I0809849

THE MUCH-AT-ONCE

AMERICAN PHILOSOPHY

Douglas R. Anderson and Jude Jones, series editors

THE MUCH-AT-ONCE

Music, Science, Ecstasy, the Body

BRUCE W. WILSHIRE

FORDHAM UNIVERSITY PRESS NEW YORK 2016

Fordham University Press also publishes its books in a variety of electronic formats. Some content that appears in print may not be available in electronic books.

Visit us online at www.fordhampress.com.

Library of Congress Cataloging-in-Publication Data available online at catalog .loc.gov.

Printed in the United States of America

18 17 16 5 4 3 2 1

First edition

Contents

Appendixes

Foreword

Edward S. Casey

However vague and difficult to describe verbally all that may be in our variegated experiencing of time, the self-compounding of the self is fundamentally real: It is at the heart of our ecstatic being. . . . The much-at-once of each is *composed* individually into a meaningful whole and sequence. That we *all* compose fugally is shared!

—Bruce Wilshire, *The Much-at-Once*

Bruce Wilshire was a great, strapping man—a person of great height and a thinker of great depth. He had outreach—into his contemporary world and its most grievous problems—as well as inreach into the emotional subtleties of the human heart and the cognitive complexities of intellect. His outsized hands wrote a series of moving and memorable books, while his dynamic body took him, every year, into the Sierra Nevada mountains of northern California. He was a native of Los Angeles, where the highest mountain in the region, Mount Wilshire, was named for one of his ancestors: I have wondered whether his own gigantism was modeled on the monumentality of this majestic mountain. Despite his physical prowess (he was a swimmer as well as a climber), he was increasingly interested in the delicate psychophysics of the lived body, finding in the Feldenkrais method (as had John Dewey before him) a gateway to a liberated corporeality. With his wife Donna, he engaged in indigenous practices and rituals, being convinced that the life of native peoples sets a pattern from which late modern peoples have much to learn.

Bruce Wilshire was a giant in the earth. He was someone you looked up to: You had no choice but to do so, not only because of his physical stature but because of the heights to which his thought ascended. He took his students, colleagues, friends, and family *somewhere else* than they had ever been before. At the same time, he brought those who entered his ambience to stand more fully just where they were. He liked to quote Emerson's phrase of "circular power returning into itself," and he himself seemed to be a conduit through which emanated a special power that enlivened the place where others stood. No longer standing himself, he is grievously missed for his mind, his sensibilities, his energies, and his passions.

Among these passions were philosophy and music. *The Much-at-Once* brings these two diverse areas of human experience and achievement into one incredibly intense text: a single bivalve treatise, a mountain of thought that mirrors its author as well as the world he animated and inhabited. It is a testimony to the reach of a man who could combine what is situated in the conceptual heavens in philosophy with the resounding rhythms of the earth in music. This book is at once comprehensive in what it discusses and wise in how it illuminates.

The Much-at-Once is a one-of-a-kind book: a book that creates its own genre. It is also Bruce Wilshire's last book. It crowns an unparalleled career in writing philosophy in creative, forceful, ever-new ways. It is a book that recasts that career, sending it in a new direction as its final gesture. But in this very regard it does what every book by Wilshire managed to accomplish: It breaks into new territory—indeed, it *defines* that territory, which is never the same after its exploration by this mountaineer philosopher. After reading this text, we shall never look on philosophy in the same way, nor will music be experienced as before. Along with these departures from our ordinary conceptions comes the sense that we ourselves will never be the same: as readers, as thinkers, as human beings. *The Much-at-Once* is a polymorphic treatise, taking many issues and topics that we thought we understood into a new dimension of understanding.

Bruce Wilshire had one of the most creative and far-ranging philosophical minds of our era. He was among the very first to see the deep affinity between the thought of William James and phenomenology, and he was a first-class scholar of nineteenth-century philosophy, ranging from Schelling to Darwin to Nietzsche. An actor when he lived in New York in his twenties, he became a philosopher through graduate study at New York University under the inspiration of William Barrett. From Barrett he learned that philosophers need to address the most urgent questions of their day and not only contribute to in-house scholarly debate. One of his most original works, *Role Playing and Identity: The Limits of Theatre as Metaphor* (1982), examined the character of theatrical performance regarded as paradigmatic for human action and interaction. This award-winning book merged his career as an actor with his active commitment to painstaking phenomenological description. Thanks to this scintillating book he became one of the leading lights in continental philosophy, an eminence he enjoyed until the end of his life.

Other books followed suit, each on a distinctively different subject matter: He managed the difficult task of never repeating himself in his many publications. *Wild Hunger: The Primal Roots of Modern Addiction* (1998) considers the issue of addiction in Western society, proposing the daring hypothesis that it ensues from a deprivation of wilderness and a lack of self-regenerating experiences that inspire and challenge us. Addictions of all sorts are self-defeating substitutes for such experiences. Another book, *Get 'Em All! Kill 'Em!: Genocide, Terrorism, Righteous Communities* (2004), approached the question of genocide at new depths that moved beyond the conventional recourse to jealousy and racism in order to find the inner logic of genocidal behavior. It shows how cycles of anxiety and disgust in our modern existence weave through our collective bodies and group symbols to trap us in paroxysms of genocidal violence.

A special contribution to American philosophy is found in *The Primal Roots of American Philosophy: Pragmatism, Phenomenology, and Native American Thought* (2000), which examines the affinities between Native American thought and classical American pragmatism. Wilshire discovers in the thought of James, Emerson, Thoreau, Peirce, and Dewey a source unsuspected in previous accounts of these great forebears of contemporary philosophy in the United States. The reader discovers that themes of attachment to the land, the power of embodiment, and nonrational ways of knowing have direct precedents in Native American thought. It is altogether fitting that *The Much-at-Once* is appearing in the distinguished American Philosophy series at Fordham University Press.

Still another book, *The Moral Collapse of the University: Professionalism, Purity, and Alienation* (1990), takes up the fate of higher education, demonstrating that the problems of the academy stem from deeper issues of self-identity and that the common sense of the academy institutionalizes a series of purification rituals designed to keep bodily and emotional engagement apart from learning. Wilshire suggests a new dialogue among disciplines and different marginalized groups to revitalize academia. *Fashionable Nihilism: A Critique of Analytic Philosophy* (2002) offers a frontal attack on analytical philosophy, above all on its reductivism. This book is as bold as it is controversial, and it earned him the enmity of many philosophers of the analytical persuasion. Their critique did not intimidate Bruce Wilshire in the least: His imposing physique was only the outward expression of a fierce inner spirit that was ever willing to do battle for philosophical thought that is fiercely attentive to the perplexities of human life.

This same spirit led him to become the acknowledged leader of the most significant rebellious action in the history of the American Philosophical Association: the "pluralist movement." Initiated in the early 1970s, this was a group of philosophers of several stripes—continental, metaphysical, and pragmatic—who were outraged at the way in which their work was routinely regarded as second-rate by the reigning analytical establishment, finding little if any place on the programs of the APA. In dramatic confrontations at business meetings of the Eastern APA in the 1970s, Wilshire eloquently argued for open programs in which all varieties of philosophy were welcome. This met with skepticism and aggressive opposition at first, but by 1980 all three branches of the APA—Eastern, Central, and Pacific—featured "group meetings" as a regularly scheduled feature; these meetings were occasions for philosophers with nonmainstream concerns and interests to meet and talk. Most important, the APA was set permanently on a course that gave recognition to the contributions of racial and ethnic minorities as well as full recognition to women in philosophy. Bruce Wilshire put into motion nothing less than the radical democratization of American philosophy at a critical turning point in its history.

At his untimely death on January 1, 2013, Bruce Wilshire left the complete manuscript of a major project on which he had been working concertedly over the previous six years. In this remarkable volume, Bruce drew on his lifelong love of music, exploring how music provides a way to experience primal connections to the earth and its creatures, human and nonhuman. Music communicates at a level that subverts the reign of formal reason. It joins our bodies to the larger circulation of energies of the planet. Music also conveys viscerally the variously entangled nature of experience, the dense character of time, the rhythms of the dramas of human existence, and much more. The title of this book comes from a phrase of William James, who wished to capture the way in which human experience is intensely held within a symphony of shared forces much wider than personal existence provides. Rather than presenting a mere sequence of sounds, music takes us into a sphere that echoes with ancient voices. Wilshire finds paradigm instances of the much-at-once not only in the experience of music but also in moments of ecstatic insight and in bodily epiphanies; music embodies and epitomizes what is possible for the ecstatic body in many registers.

The Much-at-Once is a unique creation, both within Wilshire's lifework and in the contemporary philosophical world. It sums up even as it surpasses a career that was one of the most singular in the recent history of American and continental philosophy. The reader is in for an unprecedented adventure of confronting its courageous claims and sharing in its groundbreaking visions, all expressed in highly animated language.

Bruce Wilshire was much to take in, and he gave much to the world of which he was a part. "From one to whom much is given, much is expected." This common saying (often repeated by parents to motivate their children) needs to be modified in thinking of the life and works of the amazing philosopher who was Bruce Wilshire. In his case, he to whom much was given—much by way of a supportive early family circle—was to bring forth much more than his family and early friends ever anticipated and certainly much too much to assess fully here. But the book before you will give you a lively sense of what Bruce Wilshire had to say at the end of a richly accomplished life that was lived with extraordinary intensity. He had much more to say, but in *The Much-at-Once* he said a great deal—making this book his final testament.

Preface

This book explores the world of sound, and at the same time explores ourselves, we who listen, dance, converse, sing, laugh, groan, cry out, make music of many kinds.

The ears are organs of both hearing and balance. When intently listening to the world around us, we are alert, balanced, poised—ready to move out in any direction any moment. William James coins the term the *much-at-once* to describe the influences and stimuli of uncountable numbers and sorts that rain in on us from all sides all the time. When alert and poised we are ecstatic: *ex-stasis* meaning to stand out. We stand out through our body and get caught up in things feelingly and moodily. Even boredom is a feeling and mood, however dreadful, in the spell of which we find nothing that claims us or commands our interest and devotion.

When things go well, all our senses work in ensemble. But today sight and vision have become greatly predominant, with momentous consequences. For sight can reach beyond immediate surroundings and detect things at great distances, and mind, we know, is not limited to immediate locale, for we can think about anything under the sun or beyond it. Sight and mind have become linked subtly and profoundly. Neither is limited by an immediate locale. The linkage shows up in everyday language: "I see" is equated with "I understand." Yet another linkage to what is not limited to locale emerges rapidly today: that is, our marvelous electronic communications technologies. Not even the telephone needs to be fixed in a definite place.

Let's call this *dis-location*. Because we are communicating beings, this dis-location must deeply affect who we are. An old-fashioned fact remains, however: We are also bodily beings that must at every moment be in some place. What are we to make of the new connectedness via communications that bring new dis-locations? This is not really clear yet. Technology leaps out of established frameworks for evaluating what is happening. For thousands of years we have been emotionally invested in valuing things in each other's *immediate physical presence.* The danger is that our very presence to each other—and the presence of nonhuman things to us, even of ourselves to ourselves—will thin out, attenuate; that we will fall prey to what William James calls the "sheathed in India-rubber" feeling ("The Perception of Reality," 142).

Hence the urgent need to explore hearing, which is simultaneously the body's sense of balance, of location and poise, of orientation, and the visceral presence of what might sound all around and in us, even vibrate our bones and muscles. Did we emerge on this planet through many explosive millennia to become empty and bored? I don't think so. Not if we *hear* the present and actual world soliciting and calling us, demanding a reckoning of how we spend our few moments. Am I a blessing and a brother to other beings, or a curse, or nothing in particular at all?

THE MUCH-AT-ONCE

PROLOGUE

William James uses the phrase *much-at-onceness* to describe the fulsomeness of the world that at all times surrounds, nourishes, holds, and stimulates us. But of course, "much-at-onceness" also describes the way in which the sensate human body constantly holds and processes the gifts we receive from the surrounding, fulsome world (*Some Problems of Philosophy*, 32). This provocative little phrase, the much-at-once, can stagger us with unending innuendo, suggestion, and possibility. It directs our attention to the fact that the world is much more than the accumulation of particular things that we can see in front of us. James wants us to become aware of the ever-present More-ness of the world that constantly pummels, pokes, provokes, pricks, and feeds us from all directions; as well, he wants us to become aware of the uncountable numbers and sorts of visual and audible influences and emotional stimuli that web and spark around inside us.

The superabundant, fecund, ever-creating world won't hold still to be measured, defined, and classified once and for all by us. The world is always pregnant with More, always presenting us with unseeable potential, with as-yet-unknown and ultimately unknowable possibility. We can measure and classify with our conscious minds only a part of our active, essential reality because reality must ever and always include what hovers and flows in the fringes of our consciousness, what is only vaguely perceived by us, and what will never be clarified and defined but will always only beckon to us as Possibility.

The much-at-once—the more-than-can-be-seen—hovers all around, holding us in a thick, ubiquitous, lush embrace that not only gives us our apperceptions of reality, but is the source of all our feelings and moods. The vague, ambiguous, shy streams of unidentifiable feelings and hunches that lurk and flow in the "fringes" of our consciousness give us our days, our lives, our very selves more surely than our reasoning intellect ever does—or ever can. The vague and furtive, untouchable but influential much-at-once of the world pours into us from below the surface of the ground as well as from the furthest extremes of the enveloping world-cosmos; this same much-at-once summons up from deep within our bodily being the full spectrum of possible human experiences from which our lives are constructed. That full spectrum includes, of course, the contradictory extremes of ecstasy and boredom or depression.

Let's consider ecstasy. When we find ourselves intensely alert to and caught up in the much-at-once, we can become ecstatic, transported out of our dulled and dulling habitual behaviors, moved into a state of heightened feeling, into exaltation, into rapture, into an intensified awareness of being subsumed into the All. When things go well—most especially when we are ecstatic—our multiple senses (which number far more than the fabled five) work together like personal radar screens located throughout our bodies, constantly picking up stimuli from the world, absorbing those stimuli and spreading our responses to them throughout our bodies, then sending our responses back out into the world, modified and stamped by our unique personhood (without our being fully conscious of the entire rich, webbed process or of the multiple levels of our involvement).

On the other hand, when we find ourselves dropping out of contact with the much-at-once, moods like boredom or hopelessness can consume us, leaving us empty of possibility and full of dread. When we become inattentive to and disassociated from the much-at-once of our surround, when we remain aloof over time to the stimuli and pulses of life, we can slip into such tedium and depression that nothing will claim or command our interest and devotion.

In the literate culture that many of us take refuge and pride in, sight is generally perceived to be our primary sense, able to stand on its own, not needing smell or taste or any other sense in order to function maximally. Vision is naturally prioritized in a text-based tradition—ours, for example—that is organized around reading: that is, around keeping and consulting written records about what can be known, imagined, or hypothesized. Eyes have taken on a prominence that trumps and demotes our other senses into minor or supporting roles. Especially in a culture that prioritizes controlling the environment with a sense of mastery and yielding constant productivity, the act of seeing gains predominance. With some justification, seeing has become our dominant way of taking in and orienting ourselves to the world. Some even say: *Seeing is believing.*

Over time, beginning around four thousand years ago with the invention of the phonetic alphabet and the recording of people's most important data into books (rather than in their memories), seeing gradually became associated with knowledge. For speakers of English, *I see* does not necessarily refer to particular entities we can point to "out there" in our sightlines. Today *I see* commonly means *I understand, I know.* Seeing in this sense, however, is inadequate for understanding the way in which the world holds us, embraces us, knows us, and gifts us. Exclusively visual data cannot embrace us as the much-at-once does, cannot know us as the much-at-once knows us, cannot grasp us viscerally in the here and now as the seen and unseen much-at-once does.

At no time can we *see* everything that is nourishing, stimulating, or giving us life. We can literally see only what is in front of us, what is within the sightlines of our front-facing eyes. Even then, we cannot see particular objects that are literally in front of us but are located beyond sight-blocking trees, on the other side of hills, or beyond and below the encircling horizon. Yet even when we can't see it, the much-at-once—the world, the cosmos—is there all around us all the time, beckoning to us to participate by way of gestures, sounds, and other callings.

In spite of science's desire to limit what we can know to reasoned-out, void-of-emotion, publicly verifiable facts, the ubiquitous, defiant, mostly invisible much-at-once holds us in swirling immeasurable, unpredictable currents of emotion. These deep feelings—sometimes small and subtle, sometimes sweeping and overpowering—touch and stretch us beyond our eyes' and brain's ability to catch and classify them. So, if we can't see or measure the much-at-once, how do we access its wealth of potential experience and its ecstatic possibilities?

Let's change tactics and analyze the problem differently. Let's stop exclusively *looking for* and *looking at* objective, write-able data for all of our information. More of our senses than our eyes can pick up information. All of our senses help us get in touch with the world, each sense working with but differently from our eyes. Let's begin this new tack by thinking about our ears and how they can pick up and orient us to the world that is constantly coming to us from every direction—not only from in front of us—at a given moment. We can hear what's behind us; we can hear in the dark; we can hear with our eyes closed; we can hear things at a great distance that can't be seen, like the train that alerts me most mornings at 4:00 a.m. that it is passing several miles on the other side of limestone cliffs that line the Missouri River some distance from my bedroom windows.

By way of correcting our overinvestment in seeing, this book deals primarily with hearing (an active verb), not just with sound (a noun). It is about how we can open ourselves to the much-at-once through using our remarkable ears. In particular I want to stimulate awareness of the plethora of contributions our special ears make to our being *humans* who live full, rich, healthy lives. Our ears are not just organs of hearing. Our ears are simultaneously the seat and source of balance—every kind of balance. Every area in which we are stabilized and comforted—"rocked in the cradle of the deep"—begins in our inner ears. We discover where we are in the world with our ears; they are our eco-location devices. We are bodily beings that must at every moment be in some place, at some location. Our ears confirm our location for us with intense immediacy, with undisputed subjectivity: This is *my* location. There is no need to be objective about this fact. No one else needs to confirm this fact of life for us. Listening gives us a versatile corrective to our intense reliance on sight. Listening to the much-at-once enlarges our sense of being alive much more fully than seeing does; by listening to the world, we can feel the sway of its much-ness and its immediate presence throughout our whole body and throughout the whole surround.

Much more than hearing takes place in our ears. Our gifted, gift-giving ears are vital to our being fully alive. Both the cartilaged shells on the outside of our skulls as well as the tender tentacled spirals of our inner ears are essential to our ability to gather knowledge, necessary to our ability to survive, thrive, socialize, stay balanced, and celebrate life. That we as a science-oriented culture do not focally acknowledge acute hearing as essential to having knowledge of the world is dangerous; this narrowing of possibility impacts what we choose to store and also impacts how we communicate and store what we have chosen. Since we human beings are at base *social, communicating animals*, forgetting about the vital importance of sensitive hearing to successful communication and to knowledge-gathering threatens us with the loss of some of our essential humanity. Our inattention to the way in which our ears locate us in the world keeps us dis-located. Not attending to the importance of our listening, orienting, and balancing skills—all of which are ear skills—must deeply affect who we are.

Prioritizing vision at the expense of hearing results in our present disregard of hearing as an essential ingredient in knowing. This ignorance has kept Westerners dis-oriented and nescient toward many factors we should be considering in our search for knowledge and meaning. Prioritizing vision keeps us inadequately informed, as well, about where our present habits and perceptions are taking us. Under vision's sway, we tend to think of mind as a nonphysical domain somehow at some distance from what it surveys. In fact, we are minding and feeling bodies, and we mind and feel in different ways at different times and places. If we don't grasp our early and deeply ingrained bodily habits and how they limit and shape us, we won't grasp our mental ones, and how they limit and shape us.

This book is about the aural dynamics of our surround: the rhythms, pitches, duration, and intensity of the sounds of the world and how they catch us up without our consent and permeate our very being. The chapters that follow explore the ways in which the core of our being makes music: the rhythm of our speech, the pulse of our heartbeats and breaths. Emphasis is given to the way listening develops our intelligence, how we are ubiquitously immersed in the broad spectrum of our conversing, singing, laughing, groaning, crying out, hearing the rain, wind, birdsong, rockets taking off, the music our garbage trucks make as they do their thing, as composer John Cage has demonstrated.

The word "subjective" aptly describes how we perceive the world when our ears are fully engaged. By contrast, our vision has been called the "distancing sense" because everything we see is "out there" in front of us and away from us. We can occasionally get a glimpse of ourselves—limited and mostly static—in a mirror or a reflecting pond, but we can't see ourselves totally as we are while we are functioning in the world. One cannot be blamed for feeling that the world out there is clearly not a part of oneself. When I look at the world I can feel a physical and psychological distance and difference between me and everything else. I might feel that it is accurate to say, "I am not that!" If I reduce all the input from the world to what I can take in with my eyes, my personal experience allows me to consider the world an object that stays out there and is ever separate from me.

But what I hear does not stay out there. It comes right into me, right into the core of my being. What I am hearing is, at the instant I hear it, already inside my ears, already inside and a part of my body. Sounds come into me, vibrate my whole being, and resonate with my very self; perhaps they sooth me, perhaps they make me tremble with fear, but my reaction to sounds is automatically visceral and instantly subjective. It is impossible to be completely objective about what I hear, as I might be about what I see.

Objectivity is considered the only valid way to do science and know the truth about the world. On the other hand, subjectivity is always going to be solely our own experience, which scientists consider an invalid way of getting to the truth about the world. What we hear is taken by scientists and many in our culture as just "hearsay," no better than gossip for measuring and accurately ascertaining this objective truth. Objective and subjective—will these two ways of knowing always and ever be contradictory? Learning to value ear-knowing and eye-knowing equally can be tricky.

The Western tradition continually asserts that reality comes to us in pairs of opposites: good/bad, truth/falsity, light/darkness, reason/emotion, objectivity/subjectivity, and so on. You will notice that these pairs not only function as opposites, but one term has a higher value than the other; hence, each dualism is hierarchical: One side is "good," has a higher value than the other, and one side is "bad," or at least not-as-good, and might even be associated with evil. Thinking that reality comes in pairs of hierarchal opposites is called dualistic thinking.

Westerners have long relied on these dualistic distinctions. Most English speakers see and experience them as ubiquitous and true. But as long ago as 1890 William James was able to show in *The Principles of Psychology* that the categories of objective and subjective do not actually exist as opposites, and any reasoning that suggests otherwise is riddled with erroneous metaphysical assumptions (see Wilshire, *William James and Phenomenology: A Study of "The Principles of Psychology"*). Recent research on the brain-mind at major university and science laboratories confirms James's thesis. Functional magnetic resonance imaging (fMRI), which can image a live brain *as it is working*, reveals conclusively that reason and emotion do not exist as separate, oppositional categories in the human brain. It seems that there is no such thing as a purely objective point of view (see Joseph LeDoux, *The Emotional Brain: The Mysterious Underpinnings of Emotional Life*; Antonio Damasio, *Descartes' Error: Emotion, Reason, and the Human Brain*), in spite of the fact that throughout the written history of philosophy, beginning with Plato and Aristotle, these polar oppositional distinctions have been said to be basic to reality and to human thinking.

But there is a nondualistic way of perceiving the much-at-once. Indigenous peoples do not think dualistically; they perceive that reality—the much-at-once—does indeed come to us in pairs, but not in pairs of opposites, only in complementary pairs: in dualities but not in dualisms. When one takes a holistic perspective on the world, light and darkness are not experienced as opposites (light is not always experienced as good, nor darkness as sinister or evil); both are experienced as necessary and good for life, as both give us their own kind of information about the world.

In hunter-gatherer languages, one does not usually find reason and emotion regarded as separate entities; certainly they are not thought of as *opposing* each other. They are hardly ever extrapolated from the wholeness of human perception as separate functions; rather, both are found to be necessary and good for knowing. Both terms of every one of our dualisms, our pairs of dueling opposites, are experienced by primal peoples as given together; they manifest as inseparably intermixed and irretrievably interdependent. And so forth with each pair. That is *holistic* as contrasted with dualistic thinking. Holistic thinking occurs when both sides of every pair are perceived as being a necessary part of reality, a vital aspect of the much-at-once, and therefore both are good because each has some information or knowledge to offer us. Holistic thinking begins from the assumption that knowledge of the world must necessarily be inclusive of all that is; it is characterized by *both/and* thinking rather than *either/or* thinking. Clearly, dualistic categories of what is good and what is not-good break down when one perceives life and experience holistically, finding good throughout the much-at-once, in both sides of each pair.

The Western story about knowledge has long claimed that objectivity is essential and necessary for discovering scientific truths, whereas subjectivity is only a personal reaction, and therefore not a valid way of acquiring universally true knowledge. The desideratum that permeates and governs our lives is that we should *always try to be objective*. Is this desideratum justified? I think not.

Have you noticed that when we are alert and balanced, well located and well oriented in our particular place, when we are poised and ready to move out in any direction at any moment, when our so-called subjectivity and so-called objectivity are so blended as to destroy any distinction between the two, we find ourselves *listening intently* to the world around us, anticipating any edifying, supportive signals and clues? At such times we are absorbed by and closely attending (seeing, but mainly listening) to the much-at-once, hearkening to the imprecise but tantalizing More, not broken into separate parts. In those times we experience the very real presence of possibility, which is even more enticing and demanding when it is not clearly defined. We are at such times viscerally and totally *in* the much-at-once and the much-at-once is *in* the whole of our selves.

John Dewey liked to point out the different meanings of the word *in*. We are not *in* the world, he observed, the way a marble is *in* a metal bowl.

The marble and the bowl are not changed by each other's proximity: Neither the marble nor the bowl is personally influenced by the other; neither experiences any integral kind of kinship from their closeness. The coming together of the marble and the bowl is not an encounter.

There is a very different sense of the word *in*. We and the world are both changed by our being *in* the world, and by the world's gifts being *in* us. We and the world interpenetrate and codetermine each other. Any intercourse between persons—between persons and the world that gives them life—changes all the persons involved, and that intercourse then changes the nature of the world, literally changes what reality consists of. Even a transient meeting between persons leaves a trace; sometimes a momentous change takes place in people who are only involved in a momentary encounter, but during that fleeting moment each person irrevocably leaves a part of his or her self *in* the other.

Every breath of air taken *in* from the surround changes us and every one of our exhalations goes out *in*to and changes the surround. *Interpenetrated*: That is the way we are *in* each other as well as the way we are *in* the much-at-once—and furthermore the way the much-at-once is *in* us. Each, the world and the person, becomes a vital part of the other. Each, the air and the breather, is constantly changing the other, just as each is constantly being changed by being *in* the other. Repeatedly, again and again, each participant interchanges his or her very being with the other. Over and over, the world's constant moving and shape-shifting allows no firm boundary to form around any participant in any way that might limit or prematurely define the participant self—or us.

Let me repeat: This is a book about hearing and how hearing entails a different and valuable mode of being, a different bodily reality from seeing, smelling, tasting. This is a book about how, through becoming aware of and enhancing our hearing, we can become more aware of what is too close to *see* objectively or to *know* with just our eyes. From the beginning, members of our species have of necessity had an emotional, subjective investment in one another. Our ancestors lived in the wilderness by cooperating with one another and communicating effectively or they didn't survive. Moreover, until the invention of writing, all members of the human species communicated in the presence of another person or persons; we have made all our value judgments in the immediate physical presence of and in collaboration with others of our kind. Although smoke signals across a desert or drumming in the jungle are techniques for communication across a distance, these signals are effected only by the live presence of people at each end of the communication.

Humankind's primal orientation to the world—our primal way of being—is face-to-face together in a shared home place, listening hard and well to each other. The danger of forgetting how vital hearing-in-each-other's-presence is to being fully human is that we will become so awed by our marvelous scientific achievements and incredible technologies that we will stop valuing how central our actual physical presence is to each other. Teleconferencing is a new device for promoting distance and for devaluing being in each other's presence, for ignoring what we teach each other and how we support, inspire, and motivate each other when we can see and feel each other's pulses and body language, experience each other's emotions (see discussion of mirror neurons in Segment 4, note 2; and in Appendix C). When we are preoccupied with virtual reality, even the importance of listening to our own bodies can fall out of our awareness and disappear from our concern.

Today, in addition, the vital importance to our humanity of experiencing the presence and teachings of the other-than-human beings in our surround has diminished and frayed to the point of nearly disappearing (see Gay Bradshaw, *Elephants on the Edge: What Animals Teach Us about Humanity*, and David Abram, *Becoming Animal: An Earthly Cosmology*). The danger is that, as we lose the benefits of the anchoring and rooting sense that comes from bonding with our immediate locale and all the forms and beings that inhabit that place, we will lose the orienting and stabilizing framework that comes from being with each other; we will likely lose any awareness of the human scale itself (see Kirkpatrick Sale, *The Human Scale*). The danger is that we will become desensitized to the full functioning of all our senses and the full functioning much-at-once of the world, which means being dis-located from Nature, our earth-home, and our own human nature.

One can be hyped up on drugs, stimulants, obsessive sex, or mere talk, and feel high, perhaps giddy; one might say, "I feel good." Yet in such a state of feeling good it is possible that one is completely out of touch with the much-at-once of the world; it is likely that little is actually reaching one, nothing is felt deeply about anything, and at some level one is profoundly bored. Boredom warns us: Be wary, you have ventured into insidious dis-orientation and withering dis-location. I don't think that we emerged on this planet, evolving through many explosive millennia, in order to use our senses less and less, nor to keep thinking that there are only five senses that count, with one privileged in particular. But given that this is what our culture has been training and honing us to do, I think we need to relearn the fact that listening (as well as seeing) brings knowledge, and that valuable essential knowing is sometimes vague, not always specifiable or measurable, but is still a vital, satisfying, orienting, essential kind of knowing. By training ourselves to focus on provable, measurable facts, we have consistently ignored the much-at-once and the more-than-we-can-see, with the result that many of us now seem to be consumed with juggling and caring about countless empty facts. We as a culture have become fixated on facts and data while becoming oblivious to the much-at-once and the More that contains our Possibility. As a result, many of us feel empty, have become bored, unbalanced, have wandered until we've lost our place and the pulse and music of being.

This book therefore explores the contribution that our ears and our hearing make to the meaning we find in being alive. Our ears are organs of hearing and simultaneously the source of our body's sense of balance and our awareness of our location. They are the bodily place from which our poise emanates, the place that gives us our primal orientation and announces to us the presence of the much-at-once sounding and resonating all around and in us: the moreness and possibility that can turn us in a new direction or turn us inside out, and can even vibrate our bones and muscles into ecstasy if we will but listen and hear.

If we are to change course, we must decide to make the effort to *hear* the present and actual world as it solicits and calls us from its multiplicity, as it offers us the best way to adjust, balance, and orient ourselves, as it demands of us a reckoning concerning how we spend our few moments on earth. Am I located in the world's wholeness, or dis-located? And so I make bold to propose in this book that it is *hearing* that brings us into the world and brings the world into us in a special way, a way that seeing does not and cannot. I hope you will read with ears open, with body poised, with all your feelings and senses active and seeking. I want to alert you to the fact that hearing is not only a vital ingredient for attending to your inner authentic self, for appreciating and making music, but also for appreciating and doing science (from *scientia*, meaning knowledge). Hearing is a vital skill and technique for achieving ecstasy and fully experiencing the human body's gifts.

Please read on, to imagine previously unimagined possibilities as to how you might fill any emptiness that snags you, without your seeing it coming or knowing where it came from. In the sequence of writing that follows, I prefer the word *segment* to chapter precisely because it suggests the segmental or peristaltic movement of "lower" forms of life, and indeed of our own intestines—our intestines and consciousness. Granted, when you come to this book you must use your vision to gather the data offered, but come ready to be caught up in what you hear and what you feel rising in your body, ready to be an active participant in your own growing insights into the much-at-once that is all around you and constantly changing.

PART ONE

MUSIC, ECSTASY, THE BODY

Music is the sound of life.

—Carl Nielsen

The universe sings.

—Pythagoras of Samos

Every weary one seeking with damaged instinct the high founts of nature, when he chances into the mountains . . . if not too far gone in civilization, will ask, Whence comes? What is the secret of the mysterious enjoyment felt here—the strange calm, the divine frenzy?

—John Muir

SEGMENT ONE

MUSIC, THE BODY, EXISTENCE

Music has often been called the universal language. If that is true, it must be because music deals with something basic about us human beings, and yet attempts to explain music's power and appeal generally come up short. A recent visitor from cyberspace to my computer screen claimed that while listening to music, all his questions seem to be answered, but once the music is over he can't say what his questions were.

So what are the basic questions of life? Are they specifiable? Are they answerable in the same way that mathematical and scientific questions are answered? My feeling is that the questions we have been exposed to most often—by philosophers as well as scientists and even dreamers—are those that our culture has trained us to regard as the most basic and important from sheer repetition in literature from ancient times to the present. From Plato and Aristotle's initial formulations of the highest aspects of human nature's being based in reason and the male gender, through Augustine's and Thomas Aquinas's cogitations and developments on the same basic queries posed with expectations of being grounded in an ultimate reason, unto Kant's and Descartes's further speculations, which remained firmly rooted in the hierarchical, dualistic assumptions of our ancient rationally centered forefathers, unto the Enlightenment and the endless circuitous deliberations of contemporary scientized analytic philosophy—all these variations on the subject of "what is meaning?" and "who are we?" presuppose a rational resolution. However, this reliance on reason as the solution to these questions has itself been questioned—in the writings and good sense of nineteenth-century European thinkers like Nietzsche and Kierkegaard, as well as American philosophers like Charles Sanders Peirce and William James—as a mere fantasy, a projection of wishful thinking.

What if we learned to describe ourselves more accurately than our dualistic tradition has allowed? What if we could finally accept that human nature is irrevocably connected to our being embodied and inescapably located in the world? What if we could justify shedding our dissatisfaction with our animal bodies, and at the same time shed our fruitless claims that we are separate from and better than the world that has spawned us? What if we detected and expunged the deeply ingrained but erroneous assumption that we are divided, dual beings: divided (in René Descartes's words) into nonphysical eternal minds or souls that are temporarily—only for the duration of our lifetime—dropped into physical bodies? What if we detected and eradicated the related assumption that the key mode of awareness and knowing is visual ("I see," we say when we first know or realize something). Vision is the distancing and detaching sense par excellence; the one that seems most purely "mental," the one that is associated with our minds and with knowledge. What if instead we recognized the primal role of hearing—and of moving and dancing? What if we explore the world of sound, balance, bodily movements, and become fiercely aware of these?

Our very earliest days were spent in the womb. We couldn't see, but could hear all kinds of things in cacophony or in concert, soft or loud. There was the much-at-once of what the mother heard—however muffled—as well as her own sounds: the thudding of her heart in various states, the rhythms of her breathing or gasping, the gurgling of her fluids, the sounds of air pockets moving as she shifted her positions and postures. Interwoven with these maternal sounds must have been the faster frequency of our own baby heartbeats, along with the sounds of our own body's gurglings. Some of our earliest and most rudimentary orientations were probably auditory as we floated, sometimes upside down, in amniotic fluid. Once born, our inner ear helped us become oriented, lying in a stationary position or crawling, eventually toddling and managing to stay upright, because the ears are simultaneously organs of hearing and balancing. I think if we take seriously our essential reality as bodily through and through, music will appear to be the most natural thing in the world and the most naturally explainable.

America's own bard, the nineteenth-century philosopher-poet Ralph Waldo Emerson, put his finger on a crucial fact. Music's unfoldings—its rhythmic quickenings and slowings, its joining and rejoining concordances—are part and parcel of the *body's* rhythmic quickenings and slowings, its joining and rejoining concordances. Breathing—along with the beating heart—is the ongoing sipping or gulping of life's power and is simultaneously the power of music and of poetry. Emerson writes in "Poetry and Imagination":

> We are lovers of rhyme and return, period and musical reflection. The babe is lulled to sleep by the nurse's song. Sailors can work better for their *yo-heave-o*. . . . Metre begins with pulse-beat, and the length of lines in songs and poems is determined by the inhalation and exhalation of the lungs. If you hum or whistle the rhythm of the common English metres . . . you can easily believe these metres to be organic, derived from the human pulse, and to be therefore not proper to one nation, but to mankind. I think you will . . . . be at once set on searching for the words that can rightly fill these vacant beats. (8:24–25)

Understandable it is, then, that the biblical story of the creation of human beings centers on God's breathing into our flesh the breath of life. Of course, breathing never happens by itself but only through the intricate dynamic interplay of our total bodily life with its environing world. When gripped with profound passion, we breathe expectantly and deeply; when held in excited fear, rapidly; in restful sleep, slowly, deeply, comfortably; and in dreams, it depends on the dream. The rhythms of bodily life and those of music echo, locate, augment each other. Might music conceivably be as essential to a full, flourishing life as is breathing? Ah, but why do we need music at all? Is it superfluous, a luxurious redundancy? It is not. For life itself, moment to moment, day to day, is chancy and ephemeral, and we are incredibly vulnerable in our bodily being. Events may erupt and destroy our settled expectations as well as our cunning plans. We can suddenly be broken and sucked into black holes of panic and despair.

But music! Yes, it itself can be disrupted; yet typically in the situations in which it is created and heard, it and ourselves are protected. Reliably ministering to us, it knits up the raveled sleeve of care. Merging seamlessly into a kind of waking sleep or delighted trance, we are reassured and reintegrated. Music emboldens us to think, "Yes, our lives, plans, feelings are important—not to be meddled with." Music is the celebration, corroboration, enhancement, and support of the whole business of being human. It *authorizes* us to live fully. Even more deadening than obvious despair or panic—if this is possible—is the numbing effect of mindless habit. This can be so subtly boring that it is not even recognized as boredom. For some of us, existence becomes so routinized that we no longer notice how precious are the daily essentials of life: everyday food, shelter, the air we breathe, and the water we drink and use to be cleansed. When this anesthetized state occurs, music can help us break the shell of encrusted habit and trance and refresh our hold on reality. For, in echoing us, it gives us a subtle distance from ourselves: We are no longer engulfed in ourselves numbly. As it augments us, we celebrate and come home to ourselves.

Music has always had this powerful potential effect on humans—and on birds and animals as well. Consider this: Are wolves as they howl only communicating information to each other about dangers and opportunities in their immediate surround? Or are they also exuberantly communicating and confirming their aliveness, their reality? What about birds? Are they only marking their territory with their songs, or calling out to lure potential mates? Or are they also exuberantly communicating and confirming their aliveness and reality? In the case of all living beings, in sounding our music we assure ourselves that we are not alone on the planet, that we have kin and helpers beyond the confines of our immediate species. In hearing myself, I am also aware that other beings can hear me, and I them. Sounding beings form a convivial community. A post-occupation Native American of the Omaha tribe laments:

> When I was a youth the country was very beautiful. . . . In both the woodland and the prairie I could see the trails of many kinds of animals and could hear the cheerful songs of many kinds of birds. When I walked abroad, I could see many forms of life, beautiful living creatures which Wakanda [the Great Spirit] had placed here; and these were, after their manner, walking, flying, leaping, running, playing all about. . . . But now . . . sometimes I wake in the night, and I feel as though I should suffocate from the pressure of this awful . . . loneliness. (Peter Nabokov, *Native American Testimony*, 184)

Greatly revelatory disclosures of the nature and power of music we members of North Atlantic culture owe to the nineteenth-century German philosopher Friedrich Nietzsche (early influenced by Emerson). In his *The Birth of Tragedy from the Spirit of Music* (1872), with the insight of genius, he wove together the sensuousness of sound with mind and spirit. The word translated as "spirit" is *Geist,* which in German also means "mind." So, we can ask, what is the "mind" of music? What does it distinctly know, apprehend, discern, disclose? What ecstasies are sprung? What things are sprung open?

Greek tragedies were performed in theaters, *theater* being a word that derives from the Greek *theatron*—literally, a place for seeing. For us, particularly today, seeing as spectating is knowing. But Nietzsche claims that the great tragedies with their revelations arose from the spirit or mind of the sound of music! Of course, dancing also occurred, and the *seeing* of this. But in this dynamic ensemble of the senses, it was seeing refreshed. Not seeing as the rutted, habituated, sclerotic gazing at things that lie typically at some range of fixed distances in everyday experience, with the stationary computer screen becoming ever more tyrannical (see Edward S. Casey, *The World at a Glance*, in which he contrasts fixed *gazing* with glancing and glimpsing).

Nietzsche's book discloses that the seeing and knowing done in Greek tragedy requires a living artistic matrix in which sounds and music provide the deepest roots. The music is both sounded by the performers and danced. An ancient myth is enacted by sounding, dancing bodies, drawing the audience into rapt participation and validating the proceedings. The experience uniquely discloses to each participant—whether performer or member of the audience—what it means to be a human being on this earth. This forging effect of performance is far from being mere entertainment or titillation, as it opens onto Einsteinian relativity theory in physics and in the arts (see my discussion of the music-and-dance event *Einstein on the Beach* in Segment 8).

Nietzsche believed that the high Athenian tragedies of Aeschylus and Sophocles evolved from a primal and ancient religious celebration of the god Dionysus, the divinity of intoxication, and the revelries and revelations unique to that state. The ultimate intoxication according to Nietzsche is to lose one's individuation—what makes each of us separate and unique—and to merge and fuse with the group, the corporate individual, incandescent, white-hot, living on the earth. But because each of us is an individual body that, in its experiencing, must be broken down and melted for a time, the orgiastic pleasure of fusion will be mixed with cries of pain. Nietzsche brings us, at long last, to a threshold in which strange human behaviors throughout history begin to fall into patterns and make sense. We glimpse the root motives of orgiastic wars, adulation of mob leaders, fierce homage to what is perceived as divine power, the sacrifice of self for others, or starving oneself to death; also root motives of genocide, of mutilating or exterminating oneself to fulfill some dream of perfection, some paradise of belonging. Being habitually alone and lonely is an affliction that calls out for remedy, and these activities break that encasing shell.

Nietzsche does not deny that humans typically possess powers of minding and reasoning that other animals do not have. But nevertheless we *are* animals. The power of the group presented on the earlier theater stage is a chanting, singing, dancing, crying-out chorus of primitive pre-Athenian goat-men: satyr figures, half human and half goat. Thus strands in the tapestry that are usually kept apart—mind/body, human/animal—are woven together. We humans dream, formulate, figure, contradict as no other animal can, but we often do it with animal intensity, sometimes with animal fear and ferocity.

We beings who count ourselves civilized today are, suggests Nietzsche, the thinnest crust over the deepest volcano. We love to emphasize how we differ from other animals in our abilities to speak and to reason. But also we *are* organisms with animal needs, tendencies, behaviors. More rains in on us and pounds out from us than we can comprehend—more than we can objectify and analyze into parts. We are immersed in an unencompassable much-at-once, and very often cannot tell why our moods swing as they do. The little distance on ourselves that echoing music gives us is like a foothold on what would otherwise probably overwhelm us.

The much-at-once is very often too much. No wonder we turn away from the thought of the immense dark cavity under the earth's crust and deceive ourselves with oversimplifications and airy rationalist dreams. How about our own body's surfaces and all those unseen organs inside? How about those other human-animals, those alien to our home culture? We supposedly always act for sensuous pleasure and for individual ego? What about the ecstatic pain-in-pleasure at the loss of a clearly and firmly individuated self, when the *principium individuationis* explodes and we are absorbed in the dancing, grunting, chanting group? The group reinforces, stays, and balances us. But what if it is a genociding group? Do we always shun death? What about those who run to embrace it, in love with the dream of transcendent domination—all or nothing!—suicidally fascinated that they can contribute their bit? What about the fulfilling thrill of raw contact that violence brings? Hearing Nietzsche's message we breathe a sigh of relief: Not everybody has left us to our fate, forgotten us—we strange human-animals. Somebody cares enough to listen and to look sharply at us dangling over the vast gulf of our ignorance and fear.

Evolved and refined though it was, the well-known Athenian tragic drama of the fifth century BCE still retained its chthonic man-and-goat roots, its contact with ecstatic powers of fusion and orgiastic moving, biting, thrusting, swallowing. What happened onstage with the goat-men emerged from them intercorporeally as they swirled and knocked together rhythmically, harmonically, tympanically. As each excited every other in lived immediacy—the audience also partaking of the vibrating fiery fusion, the encompassing contagiousness of it.

All this changed, writes Nietzsche, with the emergence of the dramatist younger than Aeschylus and Sophocles, Euripides. For he didn't dramatize "from the stage" but rather became the calculating, analyzing, objectifying *observer* seated out there in the audience. The "divine philter" was spilled, intoxication ceased. When the plot of the drama grew complex beyond the powers of cunning entertainment to unfold, Euripides employed the "cynical device" of the deus ex machina: the goddess Athena in statue form deposited mechanically on the theater house of the stage, who then, as divinity, resolved by fiat the perplexities and dilemmas left over in the play. With this bit of artifice, thinks Nietzsche, tragedy that springs from the spirit or mind of music, body, sound, poise, began its precipitous decline. Richard Wagner's attempt in the nineteenth century to revive the tragic music theater with his operas, conceived as "total works of art" (*Gesamtkunstwerke*), left Nietzsche soon enough disillusioned. Not even the drugged lovers in Wagner's masterpiece *Tristan und Isolde* (1859) quite escape the iron box of spectacle perceived as distant, "out there."

The twentieth century's fascination with the Mephistopheles or devil figure also epitomizes the decay of tragedies. For modern artists and audience have automatically projected the demonic ingredients of our *own* personal and collective selves into a fantastical figure "out there." We no longer deeply participate and identify with the diabolical character. We deceive ourselves. In James Joyce's *Ulysses*, Stephen Dedalus declares that history is a nightmare from which he is trying to awake. It can only be imagined what Nietzsche would have felt about Arnold Schoenberg, Alban Berg, Anton Webern, Sergei Prokofiev, Dmitri Shostakovich, Charles Ives, Alfred Schnittke, each of whom would return us to the demonic ecstasies of human intersubjectivity, which is an intercorporeality. We shall examine these figures in due course.

Nietzsche's formal education centered on philology, the study of ancient languages and their primal roots. Thus he focused on archaic or primitive cultures, their thought and their arts, insofar as they were known in nineteenth-century Europe. Growing up in midcentury, he fell into a wide and deep fascination with all things Greek, a fascination that fed the identity-building of a hitherto fractured Germanic political-geographical culture. He was also much taken with nineteenth-century science, geology and biology (though he believed that Darwinism gravely reduced and oversimplified the human condition).

Nietzsche had limited patience with what purported to be purely factual histories of humanity. He critiqued the ideals of positivism—"finally positive knowledge is obtainable through science"—as self-congratulatory and escapist self-deception. Promising to be scientific, positivism declared that *all* reliable knowing must be done by science (science as then currently understood), but since this can't be proved, positivism is scientism, an ideology, not science. Along with this came overreliance on vision, sclerotically conceived and practiced as gazing—the distanced, detached, objectifying sense par excellence—and its untoward influence on our whole conceptual and imaginative life and thought. There is more to knowing than grasping data "out there," particularly when we need to understand ourselves. There is more than what can be seen at fixed distances by the steady gaze.

As Nietzsche understood, the Greeks had grown up in the presence of the gods and goddesses. There was a god who was a paragon and paladin of reason, Apollo. Reason has its powers to reveal the world. There was also a god who was a paragon and paladin of ecstasy, revelry, and intoxication, Dionysus. These latter states—which many today regard as irrational or noncognitive—*also* have their powers to reveal things and to sustain us. They buoy us out of the static. As divinities, Apollo and Dionysus are not merely the fanciful invention of Greeks' minds "in themselves"—whatever that might mean. They disclose the Greeks' powers of identification and fusion with what pulsed ecstatically in the Greeks' experiencing as ultimate exemplars of reason and passion. These gods had their own immediate, archaic, prereflective reality and they disclosed essential aspects of Greek selfhood and its world; these chords still resound within the deep viscerality of who we are as moderns, since we live as an embodiment that, despite cultural differences, hearkens back to this wilder dimension of our being. Some kinds of disclosure can occur only through passionate perceiving and reasoning intimately conjoined.

As we will see, music, theater, and dance are indeed universal languages in which humans all over the world, even today, have similar ecstatic experiences in which we "stand out" into the world all around us every moment, and enhancements and disclosures of various kinds dawn on us. Or, if they don't, we are dreadfully bored. This is often obscured, I believe, in our "advanced" North Atlantic culture, ever more secularized and scientized. But we have our own intoxications, fusions, and disclosures, whether really understood or not in their disclosive powers and the limits of these. We have our Hollywoods, Madison Avenues, electronic games—which also of course slide into mere entertainment and diversion, heavily weighted for commercial gain, and inclined in the end to the soporific, ephemeral, deceptive.

Nietzsche seems to believe that, at a point in their history or prehistory, Greek music, theater, and ritual achieved a marriage or bonding between Apollo and Dionysus. Like many, he certainly wanted to believe this could happen. For all human cultures have discerned that we odd animals are challenged to build up an identity for ourselves out of the many impulses and powers that work on us from all sides and from within. Differently put, all have seen that we must systematically select out of the myriad of influences and stimuli that rain in on us from everywhere every moment—from the much-at-once—what is to be noticed, valued, acted upon, disclosed, and ignore or shun what is not to be.

All cultures must constitute a *world* in their experience, even though most, most of the time, do not acknowledge the relativity of this world to their own culture. No, their world is just what the world *is*, and foreigners have to be dealt with in special, cautious—or furious—ways. Thus the power of our heated, immediate, prereflective involvements in our own world-experienced; we should speak of our *erotic* and *possessive* carving out of *our* world-experienced. In previous works I have called this phenomenon "mimetic engulfment" to indicate how we are incorporated into a world and a group identity on the level of embodied, prereflective interlinkage with others.

Now Nietzsche certainly valorized the enacted worlds of the high fifth-century BCE Athenian tragedies of Aeschylus and Sophocles, but by this time the chorus circulating around the chief characters was composed of out-and-out humans, the elders of the city, who commented on the action of the play from angles not fully available to the characters themselves. Gone were the chthonic goat-men, the satyr chorus, which

Nietzsche postulates formed the archaic roots of these later, recorded tragedies. Yes, there was the fourth play that followed the typical trilogy of high Athenian tragedies, the so-called satyr play. Realizing the rhythmic cycles of human life—periods of effort, then rest and relaxation—Greek theater staged the latter plays as rests and reliefs, as farces of some kind, very often sex farces. Satyr-type beings did appear, with huge leather phalluses swinging, but the earlier chthonic power was toned down along with whatever revelatory power it embodied. The earliest Greek divinity had been the earth goddess herself. What had happened to her? What are we to make of our *bodily,* always *located* nature?

Nietzsche judged that the work of the third tragedian, Euripides, fell away precipitously from the achievements of Aeschylus and Sophocles, but I'm not completely clear what Nietzsche thought of the whole "modernization" development that culminated in the fifth-century work of Aeschylus and Sophocles. The question is important, I think, and he has goaded us toward it. One of the queries that can greatly exercise us: What does it *mean* to say that we are animals? It is one thing to dress up an actor with hairy shins and goat-like hooves and have him prance around to dithyrambic music and dance, and quite another to really ask: In what ways is a lusty man little more than a randy goat?

This is a universal and timeless question that all cultures must deal with in one or various ways, maybe antagonistic ones. John Berger writes in "Why Look at Animals":

> The loss of everyday contact between ourselves and animals—specifically the loss of eye contact—has left us deeply confused about the terms of our relationship to other species. That eye contact, always slightly uncanny, had brought the vivid daily reminder that animals were both crucially like and unlike us; in their eyes we glimpsed something unmistakably familiar (pain, fear, courage) but also something irretrievably other. (Quoted in Michael Pollan, *The Omnivore's Dilemma*, 306–7)

There is something schizoid here, or at least greatly perplexing and challenging. Is too much stress being placed by Berger on eye contact? But what are we to make of our relationship to nonhuman animals? Emerson already informed us of the amazingly intimate reciprocity between the human organism and our poetry and song. Meter begins with the pulse beat, and the length of lines in songs and poems is set by the inhalation and exhalation of the lungs.

I regard this book as a progression in intensity. The intensity is largely a matter of the tension that develops in our questioning: What does it mean that we are animals? We will find that the genius Moshe Feldenkrais discovered that the eyes—whatever else they do—are sphincters. They are tied organismically with the other sphincters of the body—anal and urinary, for example—and this radically recontextualizes and reconfigures what we mean by vision and by vision-dominated thought and behavior. As noted, "I see" has habitually become for us the equivalent of "I understand." So what do squinting eyes entail for the rest of the alive, located human body? Ultimately at stake is the question of who we *are.*

It is tempting to think that the Dionysian was a strand of the popular culture of ancient Greece, but not of our contemporary culture that has somehow surpassed such an earlier stage of cultural development; however, the rock, hip-hop, rap, grunge, and other contemporary subcultures of our current music scene are equally and plainly Dionysian. Whether in the throbbing, orgiastic, relentless music with lead guitarists massaging the instruments strapped to their bodies, or in the pulsating waves of undulating dancers at a rave, Dionysus still dwells among us. The phenomenon goes deep into the body. Often the abrupt jerking about by performers seems to simulate—present?—orgasm. Contractions of involuntary muscles are also rendered in, say, the late James Brown's ability to trigger his golden-slippered feet into apparently autonomous activity—as if they had become golden fish or excited gilded worms flopping, wriggling, squirming there on stage.

Thus confirmed is the observation of Felicitas Goodman, the exploratory twentieth-century anthropologist, that "in the long run, humans cannot tolerate ecstasy deprivation" (*Ecstasy, Ritual, and Alternate Reality: Religion in a Pluralistic World*, 171). So deep it goes! Confirmed also, of course, is Nietzsche's recognition that the god Dionysus is an archetype of human reality and will not be denied—not even in a culture still bearing the marks of Christian suppression of sexuality and of the body generally. And not even in a culture that places such monetary value on calculation, control, efficiency, such that it might devalue music with a thought like "mustn't waste much time in mere entertainment." Even if it is not apparent, the spirit of Anton Bruckner and the rock favorite of a previous generation, the Grateful Dead, have a similar ecstatic and Dionysian charge that expresses a continuity in culture in response to a deep embodied need, even in the midst of our commercial, military, and consumer-driven age.

Now as Emerson, Nietzsche, Aristotle, and many others have emphasized, to live well is to function well as the whole beings that we are, or potentially are. What hope is there today for a bonding between Apollo and Dionysus, given the realities of our electronically animated and relentless much-at-once—the huge, bony, tingling, and benumbing grip of it? In one way or another, all sectors of the human race, apparently, have felt the need to deal with our human reality, our lives not free of instinct, but not bound up tight in it either. *The Omnivore's Dilemma*—Michael Pollan's title—expresses this. How do we find and keep good habits for ourselves, say, culinary ones, and not spend our time and precious energy dithering about what to eat and what to do?

Consider China: For thousands of years "spiritual" practices developed, such as Tai Chi or Qigong—"meditations in movement." The point was to attune the body to the harmonious and regenerative movements of that Nature in which we have developed and from which we may try to totally divorce ourselves only at our peril. Particularly exemplary is the flow of water, the symbol of the flow of the Tao. How can this easeful flow be induced in our internal organs—easily overstressed—such as the kidneys, lungs, heart? The point is, through exercises, to merge our movements with the easeful, fluid, and beautifully coordinated movements of the wilderness Nature of living things around us. These ancient Asian embodied yet spiritual exercises are now being employed by some harried people in North Atlantic culture who are bedeviled by the felt need to control what is often uncontrollable.

But being fully Westernized myself, and feeling an especial responsibility to North Atlantic culture, I will mainly be concerned with ferreting out and developing resources for sanity, ecstasy, vitality, and poise that are close to home and have developed largely in the West. I am alarmed by the Nietzschean "will to power" that has broken out disruptively in our

Euro-American world, and by our rushing demonically, afraid to reflect on where we are being taken. At crucial junctures, however, I will seek the aid of Native American thinkers particularly. How might we marshal the resources of mainly the Western arts and sciences in order to avoid planetary catastrophe? Can we find resources in the world of sound, balance, and movement that tend not to be available in the traditional world of vision, calculation, forceful and cunning control—an ever-accelerating thrusting that puts us forever off balance?

Sounds that are *iconic*—a jarring idea. For we tend to assume that icons are visible, mainly matters for the distancing eye, signs safely "out there." Coins are obvious icons. They have a feel and a heft, it is true—if they are tapped or dropped on a hard surface they emit a sound—but they are dominantly visual. A portrait of a leader, a hero or heroine, are struck into them—struck into precious metal, at least traditionally. The group celebrates itself by displaying its power to establish and warrant value. The coin is a quasi idol. It can be exchanged for anything anyone wants to sell for money. Here today, gone tomorrow, it is simply used, typically not valued for itself. Only for misers or oddball coin collectors does it stir deeply and strangely; only for them is it obviously a sort of divinity, a real, if strange, idol.

But the vibratory reality of sonic icons tends to move us deeply in a way that cannot be exchanged for something else. A bugler's taps or reveille summon us as whole selves: either to sleep and restoration in the one case, or to sudden exertion and rapid action in the other. Sounds get into the body's trunk and radiate into every organ and extremity. Sonic icons move us animals, however strange an animal we may be. Henry David Thoreau writes:

> All good things are wild and free. There is something in a strain of music, whether produced by an instrument or by the human voice—take the sound of a bugle in a summer night, for instance—which by its wildness . . . reminds me of the cries emitted by wild beasts in their native forests. It is so much of their wildness as I can understand. ("Walking," 246)

In reinvolving us in our wild sources, sonic icons restore us. Funeral bells or wedding bells—the distinctive vibrations of each catch us up in the reality of what is happening. We typically go along with this; we don't just picture it "in our minds." The kinetic thrust of sound and music moves us forward, even if we feel some despair or sadness.

I happen to be thinking of the impetus in the first movement of Haydn's *Imperial* symphony (Symphony no. 53 in D Major), and of the surging opening of Beethoven's *Eroica* symphony (Symphony no. 3 in E-flat Major). The symphony is the great form, as Schumann noted, for typically it conditions us in four movements, prepares us for the four seasons of the temperate home zone, as well as for other inevitable changes and seasons of life. The great propulsive themes in Haydn, Schumann, or Beethoven are what they are because they typically end on the same note. It is as though there were no entropy at all, no dissipation of energy, as if the theme and the rhythm could go on forever. It is as if energy is perpetually recuperated, like waves on the shore ever returning into themselves to re-amass their strength.

The continuity of sound and the body's immediate sense of itself moment to moment—its kinesthesis, its balance, rightness, belongingness—is the gift of music. Our *attitudes* are adjusted: *Attitude* is the perfect word, for it does not commit us to any split between psychological (or spiritual) attitudes and bodily ones. John Dewey, the educator and thinker, speaks of the "rectitude" of organic action, an uprightness that is simultaneously bodily and moral-spiritual (*Experience and Nature*, 301). Music can be this pivotal phenomenon because it balances and orients us as whole moving selves in the whole shifting environment. A horrendous lack of balance characterizes our ever-spreading North Atlantic electrified culture, it seems to me. We are bound up in electronic networks of astonishing, ever-ramifying, and accelerating scope: e-mail, cell phones, internet, iPods, spy satellites in the sky, smart bombs, and so on. We are repeatedly interrupted and dis-located by the impulses of others, or even our own. Electricity is our simulacrum of the Greek god Hermes (the Roman god Mercury), whom we send on any errand according to whim or demand. Safely electrified, we are not hindered by—may hardly be aware of—the impending night, the cold, or the heat. The impinging environment can all be neutralized, we tend to believe.

But we easily go out of sync with the regenerative cycles of Nature that formed our species over many, many millennia, and also out of sync with our own bodies, which must always be in *some* physical locale every moment. The brain, entranced with ideas about what is to be done twenty-four hours a day, seven days a week, defies the remainder of the body. But the brain defies itself as well, for it has been conditioned and formed by Nature's day/night rhythm and seasonal periodicities to generate its own opiates, endorphins, uppers: its own rewards for timely exertions and timely restings and restorings. These periodicities are imprinted in every cell of our bodies.

When the regenerative cycles of Nature are flattened out and short-circuited, it becomes gravely tempting to import morphine and other drugs into the organism in the attempt to stave off inexorable withdrawal agonies and depression. But when artificial opiates are imported into the organism, the anciently formed body stops producing its own, and then to stave off withdrawal agonies the body-self *must* import more. The result is dependency and addictions on all fronts, from hard drugs and workaholism to sexual compulsions and consumerism. It is a grim fact that once the body-and-brain stops producing its own morphines—endorphins—this production does not easily or quickly recommence.

In Nietzsche's terms, the mind (*Geist*) of music is lost. That is, the ability of Dionysus, the god of intoxication, and Apollo, the god of reason, to bond and coordinate with each other is lost. So Dionysus, not to be wholly denied, comes unhinged from his Apollonian partner. Living as we now are, I believe, in a bastardized Apollonian culture, equally off balance—in the midst of "24/7" planning, production, control, and domination—rock music, hip-hop, rap, and other forms of contemporary popular music come as a desperately needed gasp or gulp of air.

As noted, the situation today is exceedingly complex and ambiguous. Another way to regard rock music is that it is money and trade become manic. No doubt, Dionysus *is* a god; great intrinsic value resides here. But most rock or contemporary music today is also heavy with extrinsic value. The body becomes a tool to work for capital to be traded for intensely pleasurable, passing sensations. The intrinsic value of the body itself for human existence is obscured. There is little or no time for the great emotions and moods that, like keels, stabilize and right us (rite us?) through the ups and downs of time: sacrifice, love, wisdom, endurance, quiet restorative celebration, what is valuable *in itself*. We gain these experiences only by returning to the deeper rhythms of the body to which music beckons.

Meanwhile, this demonic rushing spreads like wildfire across the planet. Decked out now in the ideology of global trade and broadcast electronically, it rides roughshod over ancient cultures and their rooted religious and artistic ways of living in Nature's primordial restorative cycles and environments. Ancient kinships and ritualized life are to be exchanged for money. Only a few remaining indigenous peoples—and some aroused Islamic populations—try to stop the crashing tsunami of so-called free trade.

Is there a music—a musical drama or ritualized celebration—that could quiet us and restore balance, poise, and synchronicity with the earth's regenerative cycles? Can we become balanced and whole? We may be so habituated in our addictive rushing that we are incapable of thematizing and acknowledging the habituation, or of working our way through and out of it. Deep habits can easily become deep trances, and part of being in a trance is that typically one is not aware of being in it.

Shock need not always merely numb us; shock can sometimes free us from cemented expectations. Ecologist David Suzuki, for example, supplies to us what may be therapeutic shock. He writes that oil exploration off the Canadian Pacific coast means the use of seismic testing, one of the destructive elements of the offshore oil industry. Seismic exploration employs air guns to blast the ocean floor with high-pressure sound waves, which are shot from fifteen to thirty-five guns every ten seconds, twenty-four hours a day, for weeks and months at a time in an effort to locate offshore oil reserves. Global evidence mounts that seismic testing interferes with whale sonar, leading to fatal strandings and the disruption of feeding, mating, and migration patterns. It has been implicated in damage to a variety of fish populations, including squid and crab (per an e-mail from the David Suzuki Foundation, April 14, 2005).

Our distinctively human capacities to create ideas and desires with our signs and symbols, and to incarnate them in electronic technologies, threaten to uproot us now from the Nature that formed us, along with our earliest human and nonhuman ancestors, over hundreds of thousands of years. It is as if we live in a perpetual windstorm of numbing technology but no longer notice how it uproots everything. We may achieve what we desire, or think that we do, but in doing so we may prevent our basic needs from being fulfilled. If we lose kinship with our nonhuman kin, won't we become out of touch with a primal stratum of our own selves? Wouldn't this be an insufferable dis-location?

Some scientists now speculate that the birds of today evolved millions of years ago from certain dinosaurs. Might we listen to birds so that they sing us into remembrance? Might the birds teach us about our deepest preconscious memories, inclinations, and satisfactions: those built preverbally into our muscles and nervous systems? Many today may bridle or scoff at this. Isn't it childishly naive to entertain the possibility that birds teach us about ourselves? Reading lines from the Roman poet-thinker Lucretius might prompt a smile, as if what he wrote long ago were puerile:

> Through all the woods they heard the charming noise
> Of chirping birds, and tried to frame their voice
> And imitate. Thus birds instructed man,
> And taught him songs before his art began.
>
> (*Of the Nature of Things*, lines 1458–61)

Beyond Lucretius's poetry, and beyond speculations by some ornithologists that birds evolved from dinosaurs, lie indications of deep involvements of humans and birds over many millennia. The discovery by scientists of the carbon-14 method of dating opens up a new vista of human history, or "prehistory"—that prejudicial locution. Our surprisingly long presence on this planet reveals a hitherto hidden dimension of our being. Artifacts dated around 30,000 BCE have been interpreted as bird-goddess figures—apparently talismans, objects of veneration and guidance for our hunter-gatherer artist-religious ancestors. For example, arms double as wings, and incised lines and shapes on the back of the objects are plausibly construed as tail feathers.

Why were these artifacts created? They probably exemplify *participation mystique*, as the French anthropologist Lucien Levy-Bruhl puts it (see *How Natives Think*). That is, is it credible to think that our ancestors adored these bird figures and participated in their power and glory? The fact is, our species has grown up in the presence of gods and goddesses—

as Nietzsche knew—and these exemplified the power and glory of the Nature that grandly overarches and includes everything. Gods and goddesses are magnetic, paradigmatic beings: the superlative makers, doers, knowers, the most magnificent and supportive role models. Isn't it counterintuitive to suppose that these antique figures, and the presumptive ritual practices attending them, simply dropped away and were left completely behind as we evolved? Can we live vitally today without role models felt to be authoritative and sacred?

So sealed off have many of us become from other living things, so urbanized and monomaniacally concerned with our species' uniqueness, it is greatly ironic that we tend to lose touch with the actual dimensions of our own moment-to-moment inwardness exactly insofar as we lose touch with the inwardness of other living things. (Think of feedlots for cattle, up to their knees in fecal matter, or chickens hobbled in egg-factories—living things with feelings and perceptions regarded as mere objects to be used by entrepreneurs.) The poet-artist-thinker William Blake reminds us of where we used to be and still might be:

> How do you know but ev'ry bird that cuts the airy way
> Is an immense world of delight clos'd by your senses five?
> ("A Memorable Fancy," in *The Marriage of Heaven and Hell*, 35)

In delighted regard Blake opens to the bird, flows with it and is buoyed by it. He doesn't see merely the surfaces of an object moving in space, but opens ecstatically to *its* experiencing, its world of delight, its being that can suffuse ours. The most primal need of all organisms—to *be* fully and to delight in this—is met. I argue that we need sacred energies of interfusion with the whole nonhuman universe.

True, we have been alarmed so often in this and the preceding century that we may have grown self-protectively numb to all warnings. "How tedious! Boring! Humdrum!" So far atomic hell has been avoided, barely, because the few parties involved have wanted to live keenly enough to avoid mutually assured destruction (MAD). But if instead of a few atomically armed nations there were, say, thirty, the chance of accidental initiation of atomic warfare would increase sharply. With such an acceleration of nuclear risk the tasks of civilizations—such as raising a family, starting a farm or business, cultivating one's individual and cultural life, one's skills and inwardness—may well become overwhelmed by the anxiety of this risk.

The fact remains that it *is* alarming for any awake person to begin to realize how distracted from our immediate natural setting we have become; how indifferent to air, running water, earth, sunlight and darkness, the manifold capacities of our own bodies always in some locale or other; how indifferent to the regenerative rhythms and vibrations of life! As roaming hunter-gatherer-scavengers over untold millennia we took shape; our needs, gratifications, skills, our very bodily shape and functions were formed: our exulting over the beauty and regenerative exuberance of *being* emerged.

Brain science has become a thriving subspecialty of scientific research and medical practice today. But we might consider the possibility that intervening directly in the brain by chemical or mechanical means has its therapeutic limits. After all, an imbalance in the brain is typically the microcosm of an imbalance in the whole brain-in-body-in-environment rhythmical, intercirculating unit—the macrocosm—of which each of us is potentially an ecstatic part. The current and fashionable much-at-once as a mad dash to produce, consume, and fend off the global dangers we have created produces rhythms echoed in our bodies and emotional attunement that destroy a more deeply rooted, interconnected, and humanly enriching balance with the world and others. Caught up in this maddening rhythm, we tend to become wedged in, easily concealing how static and stale things have actually become. A fuller and richer ecstatic relationship to the rhythms of existence are screened off from our immediate experience.

Influences and stimuli of innumerable sorts rain in on us from all sides and from within us every moment. Some come in waves. This, after William James, I have called the much-at-once. Today's physicists and cosmologists search for the Theory of Everything (TOE), for as things stand now their theories of the basic forces of the cosmos do not cohere. But even if they succeed in creating a unified field theory, there can be no true theory of *everything* if omitted from the inventory are the amazing varieties of ecstatic experiencing of which we human beings are capable.

This book sketches a unique Theory of Everything. Music is the universal language because it ministers to the most basic of all human needs: to be whole, integral, coherent, ecstatic, poised, celebratory, fully alive. When this happens, we are most in touch with ourselves and most effective as agents, most really free. We are not talking heads, brittle and bored. What resources for discovering *our music* are available to us today?

I said that we would be exploring the world of sound. By this I mean the *world,* that which engulfs and permeates us every moment in every locale—whether we are articulately aware of this or not—not merely a big object "out there." Nor do I mean merely our ears as assemblages of organs that allow us to hear sounds and also to balance ourselves. Even when we are glancing or glimpsing, and not merely fixedly gazing, we tend to see only one thing or one field of things at a time, one ahead of us and perpendicular to our faces. But when we hear, the whole much-at-once on every side, within, and at every moment pours through us by way of ears, chests, glands, bowels, and the like. These we cannot close with the facility we can our eyes. We are aurally *enwombed* in the world. We might come home to ourselves as beings who are *both* always located in some definite place *and* who have the capacity to project and to dis-locate ourselves in the far-away. We might break the trance of our current electronic technologies that, used habitually, insidiously and eccentrically dis-locate us. We might regain that long-evolved ecstatic interfusion of our lives in the extrahuman and nonhuman world—that is, regain the sacred energies that claim our interest and devotion. I mean the *womb* of the world, where there is rest but no boredom.

SEGMENT TWO

SPLITTING OF SACRED FROM SECULAR?

Things "on the ground," matters and relationships as we actually live them moment to moment, are seldom as clearly etched and distinguished as are the words we use to refer to them. The price exacted by our prose words is an inescapable simplification and staleness; sometimes it doesn't seem to matter much, at other times it matters a lot. Thus we have two words that oppose and exclude each other: *sacred* and *secular.* But when we bother to look closely at the matters they ostensibly refer to, we find that they are not neatly packaged entities, one outside the other.

As we have begun to approach it in the last segment, Greek theater does not fall on either side of the fixed, polar opposition of sacred/secular. The very distinction as we facilely use it today fails to apply to what actually went on there. The persons involved in the productions would have been baffled by our words, or what might have been their equivalents in Greek: It is doubtful that the words would have been understood. What was dramatically enacted on stage under the Greek sky was of a piece with their world as it had become their own through the ages. It was a world in which they felt—sensed?—gods and goddesses, sprites, nymphs, and satyrs; also vales, mountaintops, forests, and fields. Their world was atremble with overabounding life, and not just that which can be cut open and anatomized, or casually used and inventoried. The story is told of the philosopher Heraclitus who, naked after his bath, was warming himself at a stove when visitors intruded upon him. Abashed, they began to withdraw, but he calmed them, saying, "There are gods even here."

It is true that there were ancient mystery religions, such as those at Eleusis, a dozen miles outside of Athens. These were hidden and secret places where matters out of the ordinary were encountered: Salvific and regenerative visions or visitations were typically enjoyed, and only the initiated, the elect, were to know them. Still, the point remains that the Greek theater with, originally, its satyr chorus chanting, circulating, singing, and crying out, was a public place in the full light of the sun. In the more or less refined later dramas of Aeschylus and Sophocles, the chorus was composed of humans, the wise elders of the city, who framed, pointed up, commented on the action from angles more inclusive than those available to the individual characters. We might also say that the chorus *reminded* the audience. But with the loss of the goat-men, some depth and breadth of perspective was also lost: the ecstatic human-animal concordance—however uncanny it may be—and the life of the wild. Still, the later all-human chorus spoke of *moira* and *ananke*, fate and necessity, matters ancient and mysterious that invited audiences' piety as well as their pity and fear.

Looking back, we would be inclined to say that there occurred a fusion of the sacred and the secular, but isn't this an anachronism and a retrospective fallacy? Why think that those Greeks experienced the world in terms of our sacred/secular distinction? Why think that they could grasp the idea of a fusion of the two when it never occurred to them to distinguish them? If we perceive and describe as closely as we can, maybe we can avoid projecting ourselves back onto them crudely. Music, dance, chant is decidedly not a strictly linguistic—wordy—sort of minding, perceiving, and communicating. If we use the sacred/secular distinction at all here, we will use it only with caution.

Let's say simply that with the loss of the goat-men, some wholeness, vitality, presence were lost. The loss became precipitous with Euripides. Nietzsche reacts keenly to this; it's almost as if he felt he were being personally insulted and diminished. Nietzsche thus turns his rage on

Euripides, and even more on the figure that he discerns looming behind him, Socrates. Nietzsche's invective verges on incredible, hard to believe coming from a professor (understandably he left the prosaic word-bound academy in his mid-thirties). Socrates is described by Nietzsche as *monstrum in animo,* an animal monstrosity, one whose existence had drained off into an hypertrophied head. He is also described as one-eyed, a cyclops, implying that his vision lacked real depth, was fixated and compulsive. Nietzsche inveighs against the "rationalist" and "prosaic" Socrates.

Again, Nietzsche's intensity is amazing. He himself seems fixated and compulsive, quite one-sided. For we know there was more to Socrates than careful use of prose words, carping demand for definitions, and schoolmasterly insistence that claims be established through argument. After the inconclusive arguments for the immortality of the soul that Plato transcribes for us in *Phaedo*, Socrates recounts at length the legends of the soul's travels through underground rivers and diverse climes after death. Facing death himself, Socrates feasts on visions of his own; for example, he experiences a visitation (can we call it that?) from a woman in white raiment who commands him to make music, and he obeys. All his life, moreover, Socrates had heard the voice of his daemon telling him "no!" when he was about to do certain things. This is hardly a kind of rationalism, at least not as the word is widely used today.

But Nietzsche is on to something. Along with the nineteenth-century Danish thinker Søren Kierkegaard, he was gifted with prophetic abilities. Granted, with respect to Socrates, Nietzsche benefited from hindsight. Still, he spotted the germs of desacralization and desiccation in Socrates—what we would call "secularization." By jumps, starts, and stops these germs would grow inexorably into what was to become European civilization: science, technology, global trade, industrialization, world-sweeping commercialism, and canned entertainment—and the computer that now activates my fingertips and keeps me seated in my chair, fixed and staring at the screen for hours, weeks, months on end. In short, I mean the disenchantment of the world.

The older Greek music-drama that Nietzsche praises, and assumes, held a delicate balance, an integration and wholeness that shone and sounded brightly for a while and then wilted and sputtered out. We select it for attention because of its outstanding qualities of integration and vitality. There has always been music, dance, and theater of various sorts everywhere in human cultures, in each case integral to the situation and group in question: the gaudy martial spectacles, marches, or combats; the suasive mandolin of the later Middle Ages accompanying the troubadour's devotions to his Lady Love; the austere, inexorable chants that sounded in great stone vaults of earlier medieval cathedrals; or the roustabout dancing and singing by drunken peasants on holiday in the village square. Now, in their stead, many of us have only the sensationalism, confusion, and ephemeral violence of run-of-the-mill Hollywood movies: attempts to jump-start the jaded; spectation at its debilitating worst. We are not apt to find singing and dancing in the streets on a regular basis (see Barbara Ehrenreich, *Dancing in the Streets: A History of Collective Joy*).

Great music, dance, spectacle of whatever sort always point to a suggested but not delineated "more"—a "verge of the mind," as William James writes—that echoes the ocean, that which is named differently on the different shores upon which it washes, but is always the one mysterious whole. Ordinary, usual, "okay" music and dance are just entertaining, offering one tingling distraction after another. Great music and dance orient us in the cosmos as the strange beings that we are. Over two centuries ago Immanuel Kant suggested that all great art touches upon the sublime, upon the astonishingly huge and unboundable, upon what later commentators such as Rudolf Otto call the *mysterium tremendum*. It is that which is mightily ambivalent, escaping easy capture in prose words; that which greatly attracts and dreadfully repels us simultaneously.

The very distinction between secular and sacred must be tested, for it is particularly obtuse and misleading when we use it to try to make sense of our contemporary quandaries and eruptions. Is Arnold Schoenberg's *Transfigured Night* (op. 4), say, or his *Erwartung* (expectation, yearning; op. 17) sacred or secular? The very question leads us down the wrong path. His music is an attempt (some would say desperate) to make sense of our bodily being, our existence, in the contemporary world. Or surely, others would say, the symphonies of Shostakovich, apparently an atheist, must be wholly secular. But to assume this deafens us, I think, to what is actually opening and emerging in much of his music.

Or again, it is tempting to classify the great music of the Middle Ages as spiritual. For Christianity emerged out of the collapsing Roman Empire, in both the East and the West, and with this the far-spreading misery, dust, and fragmentation that is as far beyond our comprehension as are the numbers we have to measure the distance of galaxies and far-off stars. Clearly there was a greatly compelling need to believe that there *must* be something beyond this physical here-and-now world: something nonphysical and nontemporal beyond this putrid, poisonous, dangerous earth on which we bodily beings must live day after day, fragile, vulnerable, exposed to pain, mutilation, and death.

Yes, this is a big point. But if we focus on this urge for "transcendence" and do not listen to the "spiritual" music itself, we will miss the range and depth of the sources of vitality and insight that this music's spirit and mind reveal. "Spiritual" music must emerge from the breathing, vibrating, rhythmic, moving and positioning body-selves who participate in its creation. It must emerge from their brains, muscles, throats, nervous systems as they comport themselves on the earth. It must emerge, erupt, coil out like glinting, sharp-edged shavings from their *attitudes*—a beautifully ambiguous word that, as noted already, escapes the dichotomizing of physical and mental, bodily and spiritual. In our experiencing, even Johann Sebastian Bach's "secular" cantatas of the eighteenth century merge with his "sacred" ones, so deep is his force, his style, and his meaning; listen, for instance, to his *Coffee Cantata* (BWV 211; or read the account in my book, *Fashionable Nihilism,* of our daughter singing it).

So let us be cautious and careful. If we consider the assurances of the sixteenth-century Italian composer Giovanni Palestrina, say, sounding in cathedrals, took the form of ethereal harmonies, concords, phrasings that were expirings in bliss; or his contemporary Heinrich Schütz, who so garlanded biblical stories with notes that doubting them was unimaginable, it is pointless and absurd to doubt what so charms, entrances, comforts! With J. S. Bach, polyphonic interrelationships, counterpoint, and fugue capture the minding body totally, and so engross and beguile the whole brain-loaded and feeling bodily person that the split between sacred and secular can hardly hold—at least for as long as one hears and pulses with the music itself.

But surely, some will say, the brawny power of Beethoven places Europeans on the divide that opens out onto the secular nineteenth century and its aftermaths? Not so quick. It is easy to be beguiled by the visible surface, and its attendant facile verbal distinctions, so that we miss the deeps of musical mind or mind-body. Let us linger for a while with Beethoven's *Great Fugue* (op. 133). It was initially composed as the last movement of one of his late quartets, but it proved so difficult to play and to hear for most musicians and musical people of the day that he substituted something easier. Thankfully, the original score survived and is sometimes played today, sometimes by a full orchestra. We have better learned how to grasp it, for we have better learned to allow it to grasp us.

Beethoven's unleashing of this great fugue pounds its way to moments of exhaustion, but these give way to serene and quiet interludes of the most ethereal sort, inklings of bliss. Understandably, one might construe these as intimations of a world beyond this one, but if we delve more closely and patiently we can interpret these overall sequences of moments in terms of the elemental breathing and recuperative rhythms of the bodily-mental-emotional human race. Timely exertion, followed by timely rest, giving way to timely exertion once again, and so on, evoking the basic regenerative cycles of life that empower the earliest and most fundamental art and religion: birth, growth, struggle, celebration, decline, death. Recurring again and again, individual after individual, generation after generation, people after people—sonic archetypes, totems, icons of perpetual loss and perpetual regeneration.

The human race as we know it today, about ten thousand years after the invention of agriculture in the Near East, thinks it can defy the regenerative rhythms of the Nature that formed us as organisms, and still holds us even now, however shakily. The incidence of malaise, addiction, and frantic lives is evidence of failure, I believe. Burnout happens. The conventional contemporary training of doctors of medicine still holds sway, for example (though it is beginning to change a little now, thank goodness): a schedule of thirty-six hours "on," twelve hours "off," perhaps a hundred hours of work per week. The twenty-four-hour regenerative rhythms of sleep and wake, darkness and light, conditioned in our bodies over many millennia, are defiantly shredded. As if the point were to prove that some of the "scientific" elect can transcend "mere" Nature. I believe this betrays a sneaking supernaturalism: It is the twisted expression of a tacit belief in a "spirit" that is detached from our yearning but still bodily lives.

We can look even more closely and patiently at Beethoven's *Great Fugue*. A fugue is a concerted and ever-compounding activity. A sequence of notes is played, and while still reverberating in immediate memory, the same or a similar sequence typically is played again. In a four-part fugue, a third and a fourth repetition of this sequence occurs, and all four melodic lines are heard sounding and re-sounding simultaneously as they interweave with each other in climax. A fugue is a self-compounding, self-potentiating, and self-energizing activity.

Any fugue pertains to the deep structure of the self. Of course, then, it can deeply involve and interest us, for what could interest the self more than itself? In our actual experiencing, the present is not a "point-instant" but is elongated in time. What has been experienced a moment earlier still maintains a presence in awareness and is sensed as what has just passed. This pervades both what is directly and immediately experienced newly, *right now,* and also what is anticipated to happen. If time were not woven together one way or another for a human organism, there would be no continuity, no identity of self. This self-compounding is quite instinctive, though not always automatic (for we animal and animal-human organisms can be traumatized). What has happened is not just left behind, but is caught up, returned, retained in the processual reality that *is* the self. Bodily beings, we are habit-making, self-moving animals.

Moreover, nothing is retained by itself alone, but brings trailing after it—to the extent it can—what *it* retained, and so on. However vague and difficult to describe verbally all that may be in our variegated experiencing of time, the self-compounding of the self is fundamentally real: It is at the heart of our ecstatic being. We are naturally active and exuberant. For one's life to drag along in boredom is abnormal; drugs may be resorted to, confirming once again Felicitas Goodman's observation that we can't long tolerate ecstasy deprivation. To be sure, in a great fugue there emerge auras of what is about to come, and when it does come there is the experience of fulfillment, of fruition, not only in the music but in the self that becomes part of the music. It is a body-self that always carries with it an awareness of the oh-so-close, warm, and precious living body; so there can be no experiencing that is not colored, molded, scored by some feeling or other, and by some pulse of bodily, rhythmic, and harmonic life. The hurried and happy times; the hurried and desperate ones; the languorous and deeply accepting times; or the languorous yet slightly nervous ones—all the incredible complexity of human life just as it is lived, moment to moment.

A fugue holds things together through time. In the spirit of fugue, let us bring together all that we have said and implied so far about fugue itself. Each of us is a particular, aware, mobile bodily being immersed every moment in a palpating shower of influences and stimuli, some stinging, some soothing. This shower includes influences and stimuli that are internal to the body and that impinge on it from without, a ceaseless much-at-once. This must be an ongoing and changing constellation or configuration, with aspects unique to each individual; this is so if only because two aware bodily beings cannot be in the same place at the same time. Each of us must select out of our shifting raincloud or storm cloud of stimuli so that we retain what previous moments of experiencing retained, what *they* in turn retained, and so on, with only indefinite limits. We all anticipate to one degree or another as well. We are all enculturated and social beings, yet the much-at-once of each is *composed* individually into a meaningful whole and sequence.

That we *all* compose fugally is shared! We deeply bond with each other and coordinate this way. Various communal rituals, particularly seasonal ones, bring this home to us. As I've noted, many college students today bond through their rock concerts and their bands. These really and deeply *educate*, however incapable of understanding this some of their professors may be. Students sometimes speak of these bodily extravaganzas and self-and-other celebrations as spiritual. Moreover, unless we are actively discouraged, we bond not only with other human animals. As far as we know, *all* mammals hold their lives together through a roughly analogous process, even if nonlinguistic and more rudimentary (for somewhat related work, see Mary Midgley on the internal life of animals, *Beast and Man: The Roots of Human Nature*).

In holding ourselves together fugally we develop, to one degree or another, *autonomy*. The organism feeds back into itself, and we are self-moving organisms. Our skin is a semipermeable envelope or membrane. In that respect we resemble plants, but for us the membrane sheaths an assemblage of muscles, joints, ligaments, bones, glands, and nervous system that moves us from place to place and from stance to stance, so that *our* placement and movements can be contrasted to those of *others*, moving or stationary. This is the primitive or primordial ground of *self*, whether in certain nonhuman animals or in us human ones. The point of this book's investigations of sound, music, and sonic and kinetic metaphors is to open a fresh approach that does not prejudge how we are *animals* and yet specifically *human* animals. We find both continuity and difference. Later, in Segment 5, we will go to the American genius Charles Peirce to help us try to figure it all out.

We are "lovers of rhyme and return," writes Emerson. We are so because we are organisms. All these, human and not, embody a drive to continue in existence. We do so only if we are continuously regenerated, night and day. The lungs return to inspiration of breath after letting go and expiring the previous draught of air. The heart returns to pumping only after allowing back-flowing blood to be recuperated. We continue in existence only because the much-at-once sustains us and supports our sustenance of ourselves. We continue to live only as long as we are functioning parts of what Emerson calls the divine: Circular Power returning into itself.

We are kin with the other animals because we can all be traumatized. We can be thrown off the norm of our optimal functioning and development. If instead of sustaining us the surrounding world badly disrupts regenerative rhythms, then the continuity of our lives—our very life itself—is threatened. When waste products of the life process are not expelled, they build to the point of perhaps choking us. For instance, exhaustion and perpetual worry leave debilitating acids in the muscles. The acids circulate. Instead of regenerative continuity, there occur snarls, knots, hang-ups, putrid and stagnant areas, flashbacks to the moment or moments of traumatizing injury. The past does not recede from the focus of awareness as it finally should, but hangs on, ever tightening its grip. The new and the newly creative are pinched off. We might call this a deranged, knotted, swamped, or sick fugue.

We know instantly that we are hearing a normal fugue because the same (or similar) notes that we just heard are heard *again*, and the strands of notes at their various stages of development smoothly intertwine. Then there may occur a third, fourth, fifth entry of notes with ever complexifying and enriching interdigitation: Life cumulates, builds, in ecstatic leverage and power. We are moved away from stasis, boredom, a dead center, and become poised and balanced. We are fully alive.

The notes in a successful fugue are *signs*. They are signs of what has just happened and what is expected to happen—though only in general, for great fugues are never mechanical or fully predictable. All animals use signs in one way or another. Signs of sighting a prey animal, signs of a successful kill, signs of a destination in a yearly migration route, signs of having actually reached it, and so on. Yet again, signs made by a baby that it is hungry, signs of having found what will satisfy its hunger. In each case, these are signs of *returning* to what has proved—or will likely prove—adaptive for the individual and the species.

Evidently, some of our nonhuman mammalian kin use signs and also have some awareness of themselves using them. In now-famous experiments with dolphins, chimpanzees, and elephants, when a mark is made on their faces and a mirror is placed before them, many attend in palpable ways to the mark, perhaps trying to expunge it, which prompts psychologists to infer that the reflection is construed by them as a reflection of themselves. They needn't think of it *as* a reflection; they need only note that the other duplicates what is happening: it never happens on its own. If moving, then only moving with the habitual or master self-movement. If stationary, then only when the habitual or master is so. They must infer somehow that the other is not another being—not other from *themselves*—and all without the aid of human language. The primordial animal self emerges.

If having a sense of oneself is sufficient for being a self, and if having a body that can undergo change and also cause change is sufficient for this sense of oneself, then these are primordial selves, though nonhuman. Furthermore, these mammals can recognize creatures of their own sort and realize when they themselves are recognized as one of that sort.

Shunned animals are obviously distressed, traumatized, dysfunctional. The English towhee flaps its wings before its reflection in a window, evidently not realizing that that is a reflection *of itself.* For the more frantically it flaps its wings, the more the "other bird" provokes it to do so, until, enraged, it may hurl itself at the glass. But the mammals we mentioned make some behaviorally all-important distinction between themselves and others.

Some have maintained that while all animals use signs, only humans can sometimes be fully aware *that* they do so. Only we use signs *as signs*, and only we have signs *for* the signs that we use. For example, alphabetical or numerical signs that signify through conventional agreement, so that we agree, say, on what counts as *one* of anything, or two or more, or on what sorts of things are to be called "birds," say. Or iconic signs that signify what is signified because they resemble that. Or indexical ones that signify what they do because they are known to be caused by the thing signified, and so on. There seems to be some truth in the belief that we humans can use signs in special ways. But do we use signs in especially significant ways for establishing our *being*? It might seem that we do. What other animal could think that it refers to the whole of reality with, for example, the sign "universe"? Can other animals signify that they will surely die? Here it is tempting to insist on our specialness.

But here it is especially important to look and listen closely. Elephants, for example, are clearly aware of the bones of dead brethren and they appear to commemorate them (Gay Bradshaw, *Elephants on the Edge: What Animals Teach Us about Humanity*; see also Jeffrey Moussaieff Masson and Susan McCarthy, *When Elephants Weep: The Emotional Lives of Animals*). Can we be so sure that they do not expect that they too, and perhaps all other animals, will also someday die? Perhaps, caught up in their own presumptively inner fugal lives, they expect this sort of mortality to happen to all animals—even without distinctively human powers of thought and language, whatever *these* exactly are?

Before we go on, we must be doubly sure we have nailed down the rudimentary constituents of any self, human or nonhuman. What some have called a "feedback loop" must occur (see Douglas Hofstadter, *I Am a Strange Loop*). When a note is heard *again*, it must be sensed as heard again *for me* or *by me*. Or, if we think in terms of signs, the sign must be a sign of a specific or definite content *for me* (and probably also for others if it is divulged), whether the organism can *say* this or not. Can we make sense of this without committing the egregious error of simply assuming a nonphysical self, perhaps a "substantial soul or mind"? Nonhuman animal selves would not or could not, presumably, make this assumption, and we are trying to get to the most primordial sense of self. For humans to make this assumption alienates us from ourselves, our actual bodily selves—it dis-locates us—and alienates us also from our nonhuman kindred, from other minding organisms, for we all exist mainly prereflectively and spontaneously in the much-at-once of some environment or other. This error of assuming our supreme uniqueness has plagued the human race in many different extents and forms: We stumble around, benumbed and blinded, flailing, injuring ourselves and our nonhuman kin.

This is a tricky but fundamental business. Ironically, trying to come to grips with our actual selves, we tend to use terms that are abstract and dis-locate us. This is why I have deferred somewhat this elemental discussion of "self." I am trying to avoid the abstractness and dis-location that so easily occur, even as we are trying to avoid them! So with trepidation I now say, for any animal we wish to call a self, we must suppose it has some sense of an ever-present bodily *continuity* to which other events and beings can be contrasted. This sense of a master continuity that contrasts with the different things sensed or known by it is its *sense of self*, and this sense of self is a necessary condition for its being a self. I say necessary but not sufficient because I don't want to say that a self, human or nonhuman, ceases to be that self when, for certain stretches of time, it produces no awareness at all.

The trick is not to read the abstract nature of our talk blithely into what we're talking about. The trick is to avoid being carried away (pun intended) by terms like "mind," "soul," "self," "ego," "psyche," "the I," and so on. The trick is to avoid the fallacy of "one name implies one thing named." Even human animal selves exceed the words we use to name them. So throughout this book I develop the intuition that there is no "selfly continuity"—and therefore no self—without the continuity of the organism and its "inner life" (recalling Mary Midgley). I develop the intuition: There are no selves that are not organisms. If there are extraterrestrial selves, we must suppose that something must do duty for "the organism."

Whatever we may come to conclude about our special capacity for thought and use of signs, it is surely true that we humans can lose touch with our present and actual environments in a way that no other animal can. Perversely enough! True, whatever our special use of signs turns out to be, it is no unmixed blessing. Other animals use signs to return to what has proven adaptive for their species over time. We innovate with signs far beyond what has proven to be adaptive to reality. Our use of signs often seems to be, and is, maladaptive (I develop this further in Part II). We are organisms that, fugue-like, are deeply concerned with *return*. The young child ventures forth from the parent, but is confident in doing so only when confident that it can return to him or her. The noted developmental psychologist Jean Piaget believes that the greatest learning we do is grasping the idea of stable, identifiable, and reidentifiable *things*. Essential to this, he thinks, is what we can do with our hands: We can, say, take a lump of clay and mold it into a new shape, then we can *return* it to the original one. Reversibility. The idea dawns of a given quantity of matter, and of singular things that can remain themselves even through some changes.

Nonhuman animals without hands also achieve a "grasp" of enduring things sufficient for their own needs of survival and flourishing. Piaget may be pointing up something special in our human powers of initiative, though the powers be ambiguous. Our powers of sign-use permit us to dream up things: say, for example, our own specialness as a group that prompts us to terrorize other groups and to treat them genocidally and diabolically as beneath us, as encumbrances and threats to our really problematical identity through time. Or, we dream up an entity we call "soul" or "reflective and active mind" that we imagine distinguishes us from other animals and perhaps outlives the body. Or, we erect vast systems to account for things that resist inquiry—whether far-flung accounts of chemical determinants for obvious behavioral problems, or intricate economic analyses of straightforward social breakdowns—which ultimately amount to delusional systems of wish-fulfillment fantasies. These function to obscure realities that would be patent otherwise. William

James writes of the "unplumbed childishness of man's imagination" ("On a Certain Blindness in Human Beings," 330; see also 343).

Through human history we exhibit an understandable but dangerous and pathetic tendency to emphasize what distinguishes and differentiates things at the expense of what is shared in common by them. (We will study Charles Peirce's attempts to up-end this whole unhappy, narcissistic tradition and to suppose, on the contrary, that continuity between individuals and species, not separateness, is the more basic assumption, the default position.)

The early Greeks' dancing and singing satyr figures—part man, part goat—show the Greeks' deep and provocative insight. Without such beings, such artistic continuities and projections, we live in *obscured* continuities and connections. As a species, we live dis-located. Our technological marvels of "transcending" local environments and palpable, face-to-face bodies only add to the inherent difficulties of the human condition. We actually exist every instant in the much-at-once: we are in it over our heads. If we don't wholeheartedly participate in, partake of, the more-than-human life that can and should buoy and nourish us every instant, we shrivel up in isolation and felt aloneness. As Nietzsche reminds us, the human race grew up and took shape in the presence of gods and goddesses—and of hybrid beings such as the satyr figures or goat-men.

Nonhuman animals can balance us. We are continuous with them, for example, in that we all need to be recognized by our group if we would fully *be*. But this need can be so eccentrically emphasized in us that we go radically off-balance. We take radically appraising attitudes toward our own bodies: We dress up, prance about, make up our faces, compose smiles on them that are nearly frozen, plastered on. We often play parts obsessively and present ourselves as if we were never offstage. We can complain, as did Milan Kundera, of the "unbearable lightness of being," our insubstantiality. But we should know that no amount of regard from others can satisfy our need for a solid core of self-regard. Contact with animals, particularly wild ones, in their local environments can balance us, return us to our full selves, and even remind us of how we are significantly different from nonhuman selves.

Note well, I shall propose that the sacred is this ever-regenerative larger life that *can* permeate us totally, always. Let this be the clue that draws us forward in the investigations of this book. James uses "instant field of the present" practically synonymously with the "much-at-once." That is, we are not counting instants and placing them in sequence one after the other. The *instant* is the ever new, the complete, the always satisfying, the always was so, the ever will be. The sacred is also the mythical, properly understood, what we should speak of only in the eternal present tense. Demeter gives birth to Kore; Jesus sits on the right hand of the Father; David slays Goliath; each of us is intrinsically and irreplaceably valuable. Anything that cannot be brought back into connection with the much-at-once in our secular lives is disintegration of self, slow or fast; it is traumatic disruption of it—this is the clue I want to follow up on.

Greatly intriguingly, we human beings are both distinct from other animals and continuous with them. Many commentators think that just because we can so clearly transcend the present and actual environment in our use of signs, we are therefore superior to the other animals. Only we, apparently, can imagine the whole planet and realize that degradation of it threatens all life upon it; only we, apparently, can take responsibility for protecting life in all its forms. But equally clearly, this "transcending" of the local, present, and actual environments that must regenerate life continually is also our very great weakness. For we obsessive users of signs easily get lost in distant goals, in compulsive concerns with remote possibilities, and tear up our roots in the local. We become dis-located and so inevitably become uprooted, desiccated. The latter, desiccation, was William James's great bogey, his great fear.

It is just here that we must rediscover our continuity with other animals, if any of us would survive. Here, they are superior to us. We complement each other; we need each other. I do not mean only domesticated nonhuman animals, such as dogs, but also wild animals. To become out of touch with them is not only an injustice to them, but it is to lose touch with something essential in ourselves: It is unwittingly to hate ourselves. That is, our ancient abilities to find our way in unaccustomed places, to survive by ingenuity and endurance, to be self-reliant (as Emerson put it), to be fully alive and to avoid deadly boredom. This is the sacred wildness in ourselves (see Calvin Luther Martin, *The Language of Wildness*, a work in progress).

I want to concentrate in this book on our best use of signs, on the best in art, science, and religion, broadly construed. To be sure, there is no end to our often foolish, madly self-indulgent and self-deceiving use of signs—the Krispy Kreme life. But if we attend closely to our best use of signs, we will see that valiant attempts to reconnect and reroot us are being made. As we will see, relativity physics reconnects us to ourselves *and* to the local, as well as the larger world-experienceable in our far-flung use of signs, particularly numerical ones (see Segment 7). We will also investigate the far-flung use of musical and sonic metaphors to open up and reveal our experiencing.

But for now, we will attend to music in the narrow and literal sense. Composers such as Arnold Schoenberg and Alfred Schnittke locate our dis-locations in their music. Much music from the early twentieth century through to the twenty-first conveys that we do not feel at home in the world. What strange animals we are! We humans have always been creatures of our cultures' use of signs of all kinds. The human species has had to make itself at home in the world to a degree unknown to other species. But now we live in vast cultural disruption: Things are changing so rapidly that our conceptual frameworks for evaluating what is happening—built up in the past—cannot keep up. We might speak of a cultural trauma that is also, inevitably, a trauma for each of us.

The continuities and bondings of music—and its most intimate companion, dance—reinforce and protect us somewhat against the inevitable disruptions of life. That is, the chanciness, the traumatizing shocks of intrusion, the threats of aloneness, the despair when the fundament drops out from our being: when we are filled with that all-consuming feeling that the sun will never rise again, that there will be singing and dancing no more. Of course, music is concerned not just with bright visible things but also with "the close and holy darkness" (as Dylan Thomas puts it in the closing line of "A Child's Christmas in Wales," 1952) as it is directly heard and felt; when trust is unquestioned and refreshment is deeply and instinctively expected, as when we slide easily and trustingly into sleep, for instance. The innards of our bodies move and develop in close and holy darkness.

It may be that music, in its singing and sounding, weaves itself into our lives, making them bearable for us even under the blackened sun of schizophrenic states or episodes. For when auras of these are suggested or anticipated by music, they become sufferable. It is a chief virtue of Schoenberg and other twentieth-century composers to sound our full selves into ourselves, taking even those darker disruptions of our normal rhythms and giving them back to us in a music that makes living more tolerable for us bodily-mental-emotional-spiritual beings. Indeed, the virtue of their music is to make even the apparently paradoxical nature of our human lives evident and bearable, maybe even strangely ecstatic and ennobling!

Let us take a step back and recenter on Beethoven for a while. He felt the numinous power of freedom and of agency. He initially dedicated his *Eroica Symphony* to Napoleon, for he thought he found in that man the incarnation of freedom, liberation from old shackles. (Notice how the opening theme of the symphony returns confidently to the starting note of Beethoven's only opera, *Fidelio.*) But when Napoleon crowned himself emperor and became another tyrant, wild for conquest, Beethoven expunged the dedication, replacing it with "To the memory of a great man." Freedom has a depth that even Beethoven could only attempt to plumb in his very last works (see also the later works of philosopher F. W. J. Schelling).

Many nonetheless still hunted for "the great man," whoever or wherever he might be, but we cannot say that Anton Bruckner, toward the close of the nineteenth century, was infatuated with any shining heroic human figure or with any easy infinite (earlier Kierkegaard, in the middle of the century, identified the grave danger of the false infinite). Bruckner heard the vast ocean. The great Austrian composer and organist, a Catholic mystic, dedicated his ninth and last symphony "to the beloved God, if he will accept it" (Symphony no. 9 in D Minor, unfinished). On his deathbed, though once complaining of a "clouded" mind, he worked on the last movement, projecting a culminating fugue that was never completed (he challenged himself with a fugue that moved from a four-bar one to a three) and composing revolutionary progressions, climaxes, recapitulations, and mighty dissonances. These latter the conductor Nikolaus Harnoncourt brilliantly attributes to Bruckner's sense of the divine: the *mysterium tremendum,* that which both attracts through our adoration and repels through our dread of its power. The divine can only find expression, that is, in tremendous dissonances and contradictions.

But surely this is sacred music? Ah, we should be cautious in plastering on that word. Though it would pain the devout Bruckner to say so, the divine he conveys to us is open to question and to expansion beyond its Christian rubrics. Frequently, the massive symphonies open with a mysterious tremolo, as if we were caught up in some strange and awesome birth: the birth of the universe insofar as we can experience it and commemorate it in the art of sound? Bruckner's deliverances, I believe, are compatible with pantheism of certain varieties, or better yet, with a sense of Nature as the sacred that *no* traditional Western institution has formalized—which is one central reason for attending to Native Americans.

But so incapable were Bruckner's students—and the age—of comprehending what he was doing that some students are thought to have given away pages of the autographed score after his death as mementos or "devotional objects" (some musicians speculate that the gaps in the score are most plausibly explained as missing whole pages). Harnoncourt assembles the fragments of the Ninth's last movement and declares them "like a stone fallen from the moon" (see Harnoncourt's talk on the first CD of the recording). Here is an icon that commands attention! Utterly incapable of comprehending what the devout and mystical Bruckner was doing, and not knowing or caring enough to try, the Nazis set him up as a fascist hero of power and glory: a pastiche, plaster-of-Paris Bruckner. Hannah Arendt is right, isn't she, to speak of "the banality of evil" (see *Eichmann in Jerusalem*)?

Life is so contingent, so daily, as a James Joyce character puts it. With the rise of seventeenth-century natural science and its intimate companion, modern technology, Europe had passed through a fateful transition. The book of Nature is written in mathematical characters, said Galileo, and mathematics was no longer conceived by him as integrally related to music, religion, and the practice of life. It had been thousands of years since the Presocratic Greek mystic and mathematician Pythagoras lived, and Galileo did not—could not—try to retrieve him. The world had changed too much: The world was only dead matter, basically, and this was diced up through atomist-based mathematics and was disenchanted, desacralized.

Of the so-called Western religions, only Islam, flourishing mainly outside Europe, did not pass through this desacralization of Nature. Only Islam never experienced in such a dire way what we call the splitting of the sacred and the secular. Now North Atlantic military, commercial, and entertainment power roll heavily across the earth and excite to fear and rage Islamic militant fundamentalists. They consider it their God-given duty to exterminate us, for we poison and destroy their ability to hold their lives together ecstatically through time, to live as devout agents, as selves-under-God.

Music holds pride of place in this book, in this account of strands to be woven, but of course there is danger in this. That is, that we will think that we can understand music "in itself," and then say that science, ecstasy, the body are "like" it in certain respects. Thought about this way, music would be *proton analagon* (first principle) in traditional language; it would be the irreducible basis from which other things are projected as "like" it in certain respects.

This would be a highly seductive and disastrous course, I believe—seductive for two main reasons. First, ever since the momentous rise of seventeenth-century science, deeply marking and shaping our experienced world, it has been assumed that the only effective mode of inquiry has been mechanistic-scientific—or positivistic—and that this builds an understood whole only out of simple, irreducible parts. The parts are "atoms" of some sort, a word borrowed from the Greek meaning *unsplittable*. The atoms may be those material entities, too tiny to be directly observed, the "atomies" of which John Locke wrote, and which he assumed must be supposed. Or they may be unsplittable and irreducible "mental entities," of which René Descartes spoke, and assumed them to be irreducible *supposita* (sensations, simple ideas, etc.).

The second main reason for this seductiveness stems from the traditional schoolmasterly insistence, "Define your terms!" that has terrified so many of us when we were young. But as William James and other "pragmatists" pointed out, when this happens prematurely we get premature crystallization, and this blocks the road of inquiry and the burgeoning development of thought, learning, inquiry as nothing else can. (Edward Gibbon, in *Decline and Fall of the Roman Empire*, depicts a comparable phenomenon when he observes: "A cloud of critics, of compilers, of commentators darkened the face of learning," 46.)

The grave danger is to assume that music is organized sounds, and that sounds exist in themselves as atoms. But this is to be possessed by reified words and abstractions before we know it, abstractions we accept normally and innocently and intelligently enough, it no doubt seems, but abstractions that have lifted sounds out of the *actual sounding world* around us, in which they make sense to us. There are no sounds in themselves, atoms, but things along with other things that are *sounding for us* experiencing bodily beings. (The notes inscribed on a music score are signs for such sounds, for those who can read them.)

The same warning applies to the supposed formal components of musical sounds: harmony, rhythm, melody, whatever. Defining them ab initio easily leads to that hyperspecialism and desiccated academicism lamented by Emerson, Nietzsche, and the pragmatists—that is, leads to that fragmentation in which we are so many "walking monsters": a finger, an ear, a forehead, but never a whole person. We and our musics have lost our lives. (Thus apprehensive about the seductive power of visualism and mentalism, I refrain from offering printed musical scores and notations.)

So should we ab initio define "ecstasy" too? What if we went to the Greek *ex-stasis*, meaning "to stand out from and into," as pointed out already in my preface. And what if we found that only by standing out and into the whole world experienced can we be whole individual beings? But what would we have really gained in terms of concrete and vital meaning? And what would we have lost? More than we imagine, most likely, given that well-propelled, greased, molded, routine verbal abstractions satisfy us too easily. We will really have lost the concrete reality, the much-at-once of the finite, situated, sited, experiencing, bodily beings that we *are*. We will have easily slipped into the abstracted, objectifying—visually dominated—gazing and fixated view of our bodies as objects only. Which is not as we actually live them moment to moment, for we live them as who we ourselves really are, that is, as acting, pulsating, rhythmical body-subjects (to use what is itself a troubling locution, but not the worst of the worst).

We have already cited Emerson's revealing observation that the structures of music fit the structures of our living, breathing, pulsing bodies—our rhythmic and harmonic bodies. Music is the aptly termed universal language because human bodies worldwide are more similar to each other than they are different. In another essay, Emerson writes of painters absorbing themselves in the movements of children, and then having this absorption flow out spontaneously and melodically in their painting of them. The latter adverb—*melodically*—has meaning because, he says, "the soul of the thing is reflected by a melody" ("The Poet," in *Nature and Selected Essays*, 273). "Soul" is kept palpable, tangible, evident, bodily, rather than being a reified abstraction for some alleged entity that one may speculate survives the body's death. "Soul" in its concreteness means the feeling, experiencing, perceiving bodily being whose subjectivity must be understood in spatiotemporal kinetic terms, and that exhibits that continuity that allows it to contrast with the continuities of other beings, that allows it to be a self.

For example, when a melody of movements ends in an emphatic *up* position, what is probably conveyed is the body-self's alertness and energy, its being prepared to deal with whatever comes. But, of course, even this may be too atomistic, too much isolated from context to convey the concrete reality we live immediately, moment by moment in locales. This reality is the whole interrelated, moving matrix of things and events, the much-at-once in which we live involved and embedded, but which we can talk ourselves out of—sort of.

We must even be careful with the idea of the fugal, what I take to be a central point in laying out the nature of music and self. To use the older language, the fugal is a *species* of a larger *genus*, *simul in multis*: that is, the same or the similar in the many different things or events. It is the clue to how we organize a whole *world* in our experience—including the self, of course. To talk of the fugal structure of the self is to pick out but one manifestation—however central—of the same in the different. Other manifestations may be subtler. Say an emotional tonality that runs through a symphony. Even a scherzo that would be naively or hurriedly described as "up," playful, rollicking, may be actually heard as a reaction-formation to a heavy undercurrent, a depressive mood: for example, the scherzo movements of some of the great Shostakovich symphonies, such as the sixth.

Which recalls us to the sex farces in Greek theater. These are not meant to stand alone in our experience, but to be witnessed as relief from the tragedies. The theater and the dance: key ways of keeping our account of music concrete, integrated, rooted in actual life, an element animating that whole life ecstatically—perhaps we can also say, sacramentally? To recall, I mean, that systematic courting of spontaneity, that courting of energy-exchange between many and various beings.

Earlier in this segment—caught up in Nietzsche's thought—I referred to the Greek tragic theater as dealing with matters ancient and mysterious. Schematically put, for the moment, the sacred is what is supremely, unqualifiedly, valuable. It endures. Tragedy emerges from the spirit or mind of music because the sounding of music evokes what is lasting or enduring, and it evokes it in the most involving—moving—way. That is, it does so for us beings in our first-person experiencing reality—both in our singular and plural first-person experiencing reality.

Evolution has seen to it that we are singular organisms whose sense-modalities are "designed" to work in the most intimate ensemble. We need all our senses working together, complementing each other. Vision is particularly essential for vulnerable beings such as ourselves who cannot measure up to certain other animals in terms of speed, muscular power, tooth and claw armaments, balance, or auditory and olfactory acuity. Vision enables us to identify individual beings at a distance and to keep track of them as they move in space and time. We can identify at a distance various sorts of valuable or dangerous creatures, as well as individual instances or members of those sorts. For example, "That tiger there—with the long scar across its face?—he's gotten a taste for human flesh and blood and is very dangerous."

Trouble began for us, however, when the great importance of vision became emphasized at the expense of other sense modalities, becoming the paradigm for both sensing and knowing—most noticeably since the advent of seventeenth-century science, technology, and industry. Sound stretches itself out in time, whereas a visual glimpse of something—though perhaps momentously important—is momentary. For an illuminated surface to endure as lit, the source of the light must endure also (setting aside for the moment fireflies, phosphorescent minerals, and certain self-illuminating sea creatures); however, *sounding* bodies can resonate or resound (re-*sound*) after what caused them to sound has ceased.

Momentariness—the *now* understood as an atom-moment—has spread across and deep into current North Atlantic culture. The short-term has eclipsed the eventual, and certain immediately apparent visual characteristics of persons have eclipsed their deeper and inner features: their actual ways of experiencing the world, who they *are*. Consider the glossy magazines at supermarket checkout lines featuring photos of celebrities. These celebrities are projections of our own sins-of-the-poseur, our own sputtering efforts at gaining recognition, probably our own inner emptiness: they provide a glossy vicarious image of existence, allowing us to evade the depths of who we are. Contemporary culture is benumbed and besotted with celebrities. It is nearly the worst entrancement, as people thus entranced keep themselves distracted from their own typically unfulfilled lives.

Since it is the very nature of the self to retain its identity through time, to stretch itself out through many different moments *simul in multis*, it becomes clear why Nietzsche insisted that Greek tragedy arose from the spirit or mind of music. Yes, this included of course visual spectacle, the ability to track in space and time particular characters "out there" on the sun-drenched stage. But to grasp a character's development as a person and, along with this, the development of a dramatic plot toward its fruition or telos, music and dance were root essentials.

The sacred is what retains its significance for human beings; it endures because through it we bond over time and space with the whole enduring community of beings without which we could not exist at all. It is likely that we share with animals their olfactory—sniffing—ways of building up a world in our experience, identifying groups and individuals as the same over time, but our olfactory abilities seem to be declining through lack of use. Widespread use of smart phones and other portable technologies will further diminish this olfactory faculty for navigating vitally and fully through the world and will very probably cause us to miss that anything is missing. It will also, ironically, diminish the power of sound, for this power is a matter of gathering for ourselves here and now the power of what endures through indefinitely many heres and nows, indefinitely many much-at-onces.

This here and now in its felt coherence and concrete multiplicity is held together—whether acknowledgeably or not—only through the bonds of the sacred, *simul in multis*. As Thoreau put it in *Walden,* "Be it life or death, we crave only reality. If we are really dying, let us hear the rattle in our throats and feel cold in the extremities" (92). What a refreshing change from being incessantly battered by the ephemera that issue from our newfangled electronic technologies! It is when we are not arbitrarily and artificially dividing the sacred from the secular, nor caught up in prosaic words or flashing images, that we are most vitally in touch with ourselves, most vitally alive, most truly free. That, as far as I can tell, is the truth. But it must be more fully unpacked; otherwise it itself will be too abstract and schematic.

So we need to open out new attempts to make ourselves feel at home in a world that changes dazzlingly fast. We are not machines in which stimuli are pushbuttons that generate fixed responses. We are more or less autonomous organisms sheathed in semiporous membranes that can take in whole situations. We are cultural-animal beings living forward into the light and into the resonance of our future. We need not be frozen in detached third-person objectifications. We can be up to the immediacy of the much-at-once, up to and equal to the call of first-person attitudes and approaches: a first-person that is both singular and plural.

Imagine again the Athenians in their theater under the sky and sun, hearing the chanting of their choruses, recalling their legacy as a people. We have backing us up the legacy of the human-animal species. We can choose. Our human ability to create meaning is never predictable or determined. At moments we can abandon calculation, as Emerson put it, and allow spontaneity, the divine, the sacred to have their way with us. As Schelling observed, we never escape the site of our freedom. This is our special burden *and* opportunity as humans, as the distinctive organismic selves that we are.

SEGMENT THREE

WHERE ARE WE? LOCATIONS AND DIS-LOCATIONS

Body am I, and soul, thus speaks the child . . . but the awakened and knowing say: body am I entirely, and nothing else; and soul is only a word for something about the body. . . . "I" you say and are proud of the word. But greater is . . . your body and its great reason: that does not say "I," but does "I."

—Friedrich Nietzsche

Amidst revolutionary outbursts, creative forces of Europe in 1800 were aglow with self-assurance. Technologically, commercially, militarily outfitted, Europe aimed to colonize and to subjugate the world. Dynamic expansion was in the air: G. W. F. Hegel called Napoleon the World Spirit on horseback and declared that Europe was the goal of history. He was not overly impressed with Islam. Meanwhile, the evolving aggregation of colonies in North America stamped their newfound authority in coins bearing the portrait of a heroic George Washington: "Unity States of America," 1783. The United States was a breathtaking and suspenseful adventure in nation building: the Experimental Nation. Properly educated, could we—with struggle—govern ourselves according to principles of reason? Theocracies were unnecessary, it was believed. Revolutionists pledged their *sacred* honor in creating this nation. (I will continue to trace the course of this careening national experiment in Segment 6.)

This vibrating reality, this spirit in the air, is caught and augmented in the driving, dynamic music of the early and middle Beethoven. His *Great Fugue*, though composed quite late, is a particularly overwhelming version of it. As he aged and his deafness closed in on him, Beethoven explored byways of the self, its infinitely varied feelings, moods, glimpses, inklings. The body-self could stretch itself over more differences, around more corners, and through deeper crevices than could easily be imagined beforehand. Late in his life, Beethoven exhibited a sort of self-assurance much different from that found in his earlier work and in the age as a whole. How strange and various was the human self that he explored! His last compositions baffled most of his contemporaries, and if he hadn't been famous, and well known as a moneymaker, his last music would not have been printed and published. Franz Schubert was not so fortunate: his great, and greatly disturbing, last string quartet was not published during his lifetime.

European conquests continued through the nineteenth century and into the twentieth, but without the blithe and heady self-assurance of the early 1800s. Revolutions continued on every level of human existence: civic, political, economic-technological, intellectual, scientific, artistic, emotional. Biologist Charles Darwin connected our species with nonhuman forms of life; psychoanalyst Sigmund Freud opened the pit of the subconscious body-self; economist and philosopher Karl Marx exposed the crushing inequities of capitalist industrialism and colonial world trade. The very reach and success of colonizing brought back to thoughtful Europeans modes of thinking and living greatly different from the European: Indian and Chinese Buddhism, Taoism, Japanese Shintoism and ancestor worship, many different North American indigenous conceptions of "the great mystery"—for example, Wakan Tanka—and I do not forget the animism brought directly from Africa by the slaves. These ways of constructing worlds in experience diverge dramatically from the traditional European.

The philosopher Martin Heidegger discerned, "The nineteenth century—still the darkest of all the modern centuries up to now" (*Off the Beaten Track*, 75, translation emended). Dark and pregnant, that is, with the future; dark with half-uncovered possibilities; dark with portent and uncertainty and overbrimming with bewildering pluripotentiality.

"Romantic" has become a byword for sentimentalism and escapism. The root of the word, *roman*, reveals the new, the novel; for the Romantics it connoted renewal. In 1800, world conquest was Nature conquest. This amounted to utter disruption of seasonal and localized rites that had ordered traditional human societies and peoples day to day, season to season, generation to generation for untold thousands of years. This meant that the ability to construct a world in experience was disrupted, which meant that the ability to construct an identity in both individual and group was also disrupted. Needless to say, the traditional experience of the sacred was blunted or shattered. But we humans have to look for ways to construct a *world* in experience—that is, a whole of things that endures through time and maintains its master identity. Otherwise *we* cannot endure and *be*, and to be is the deepest of all possible needs. We must feel and believe ourselves to be real and potent—to be effective agents of change, and to be really continuous and alive through time. This urging and tendency may become greatly wayward.

In Beethoven's famous earlier music, as contrasted with the late, there appeared a framing, a clear posing of self as courageous, magnanimous, serene, fulfilled, as finally above the battle, or similar. There emerged objectification of the self as it wants to be viewed by some valued observer. There also appeared the corollary: objectification of how the opponent-viewer of the self is to be regarded, the ultimate one being the devil, the Great Demon. But atonal music and its world, emerging around 1900, brings no such unrolling of a tale of struggle and resolution. There are demonic elements, to be sure, but they are relentlessly bubbling and fetid ingredients of *our own* easily troubled, ambiguous, inescapably bodily selves and lives. Without feeling at home in the world, the self begins to flake away into the void. It tries to save itself in the arts and sciences. Atonal music aims at both containing and conveying this flaking away into the void.

The dynamic drive of the Enlightenment toward the to-be-amassed, the to-be-disclosed and achieved—heard in early and middle Beethoven—is replaced in the later nineteenth century with something quite different in Bruckner. No longer does the bustling Napoleonic dynamic of conquest sound, nor do the clanging instruments of industrialization and mastery. Though no great artist or scientist tries to imitate or just mechanically return to the past, Bruckner does recall the premodern Christian world of medieval chant and, later, Palestrina. Clearly, the message is that we have already arrived; it is only a matter of opening to this eternal reality and source and acknowledging it. We already float in the ocean of divinity out of which we have somehow emerged. The old Creation myth resounds, considerably transfigured.

The time integral to Bruckner's music is more cyclical than linear. The music very often begins, as earlier noted, with a premonition of a mysterious birth. For us, this is our emerging realization of what has always already been with us—the mysterious universe itself, that which is beyond our ability to comprehend why it exists at all. The climax of the symphony usually sounds right off, and may soon lapse into silence, as if a wave of an everlasting sea, having broken on the shore and raced up onto it, retreats into the belly of the water to recuperate itself at its own speed, to re-collect its power to break again and again on the shore. The connection with Emerson is not accidental. A spiritual hunger roams about for satisfaction.

In the silence lies the fecund darkness. Darkness joins light as jointly revelatory and necessary. Darkness pertains to the interior body—that of the individual and the group, or corporate individual—and also to the body of the earth, cycling in the heavens and permeating all us organisms with its regenerative harmonies and rhythms. We are permeated even as we human organisms, with our distinctive ideas and manias to control, attempt to "free" ourselves from Nature's enlivening rhythms, for they have structured every cell of our bodies. As if trying to live in a perpetually benumbed and entranced "jetlag," we crave stimulants, soporifics, or various addictive drugs. The mind of music embodied in Bruckner moves to restore us to our deepest source, though calling it "nature mysticism" is more misleading than informative.

There had been night music during the Enlightenment, or *Aufklarung* ("clearing up" in German)—Mozart's famous divertimento *A Little Night Music* (Serenade in G Major, K. 525) comes immediately to mind—but it is brilliant diversion and entertainment as its rhythm and tone seems to skip lightly over the surface of things. Or, perhaps, the troubadour's mandolin-accompanied night songs for his lady love might come to mind, but troubadours followed an established protocol, an elaborate local tradition. For Bruckner, by stark comparison, darkness and silence probe and search for the ground of our being. This tendency also occurs in a kind of turmoil in Gustav Mahler. In both these composers there are many dark, sustained, turbulent episodes that finally break forth into sweeping and redemptive-sounding passages.

In contrast to the usual sonata form that appeared in eighteenth- and nineteenth-century symphonies, in which two themes juxtapose themselves and interact dialectically, Bruckner typically features three themes, which are, moreover, often divided by silences. His themes are more like icons—or better, more like great gestures—within some well-established but mysterious religious service. The last movement of his Fifth Symphony opens, as does the last movement of Beethoven's Ninth Symphony, with repetitions of the main themes of the preceding movements. But unlike Beethoven's—which moves toward the "new song," the choral anthem of *Ode to Joy*, an ecstatic tribute to the promised brotherhood of man—Bruckner's summons to fruition the orchestral resources already deployed in the symphony, almost as if we were commemorating the sacredness of the mysterious birth of the world that occurred long, long ago—once upon a time. In its undiminished reverberations we continue to live, move, and have our being, however distressed it is. The cosmic birth is not left behind. Time is more cyclical than linear. "There is never a beginning, there is never an end . . . but always circular power returning into itself" (Emerson, "The American Scholar," in *Nature and Selected Essays*, 85).

The orthodox Christian account of the world is simultaneously the most linear and the most heroic: God creates the world ex nihilo and drives and directs it to the "last days," to the resurrection of the elect somewhere removed from the face of the earth, when time and space will be no more. Approached from this angle, we would have to say that Bruckner is not an orthodox Christian.

To be sure, in much of late Beethoven we experience the strangely personal and private, yet that which can also be construed as commemorating the most mysterious, all-encompassing, more-than-merely-personal births and ecstasies; for example, the last movement of his final piano sonata (no. 32 in C Minor, op. 111, with notable performances recorded by Artur Schnabel, Clara Haskil, Arturo Michelangeli, and Anatol Ugorski) stretches itself to generate and encompass organically many great differences and modes: It is *sacred* music in some important but elusive sense. *Simul in multis.* Even jazz is anticipated in the pivotal moment of the last movement.

Bruckner's distant student Gustav Mahler appropriated the master's darkness for his own purposes of exploration. The question of the sacred becomes highly experimental and problematical. There is distinctive wisdom to be sought in darkness, and in encompassing and composing that, but we are left with grave questions. No accident that Mahler's music is contemporaneous with the revival of interpretation of dreams by Freud and Jung (note particularly the Seventh Symphony, *Song of the Night*, in E Minor).

With Mahler, we are not much tempted to slap the label "sacred" onto the music. Time-honored dualisms and oppositions do not apply with certainty. Simplifications such as the binaries *A* and *not-A*, where if one is not the case, the other must be. Dualisms like light versus darkness; fact versus fancy or fiction; God versus Satan; natural versus supernatural. Oppositions like good versus evil; domestic versus foreign; beginning versus ending; waking versus sleeping. At the very most, we might fancy this music to be sounding a kind of pantheism: All is divine, although the meaning of that is highly problematical. We are kept probing, ecstatically, for more and more meaning.

Even when we hear gross allusions to Nature, as in the sound of cowbells in a Mahler symphony, it is far from clear what it all means. The composer invites us to grope for meaning. True, we can regard this music as related to the Romantics' warnings that the ever-accelerating industrial age, with its varied revolutions on every hand, has lost its roots in the Nature in which our species was formed, and that we are burning ourselves out in frantic activity. But Mahler poses questions and difficulties without offering clear resolutions. It is as if he were trying to awaken us rudely from what the cultural historian Thomas Berry has called the technological trance (see, e.g., Thomas Berry, *The Dream of the Earth*).

This scenario was broached earlier in the nineteenth century by Richard Wagner. His four-part cycle of operas, *The Ring of the Nibelungs*, develops a heroic myth of the struggles, aspirations, and sacrifices of humans and humanlike gods and goddesses. The twilight of the divinities and the burning down of Valhalla or heaven is certainly significant for the age. But Wagner interrupted his composing of his third opera in the cycle, *Siegfried*, to embark on a deeper and much more ambiguous venture. That is, the tale of the drugged lovers in *Tristan und Isolde,* which is ushered in by a portentous innovation: The first three notes compose the aptly termed infinite melody; it promises *no sure return* of the hero and heroine to home, no sure resolution of dilemma or quest. And indeed, the opera holds none.

More than one of the earlier Romantics had sighed and sung, "Oh my Greece, you shall live again." By the close of the nineteenth century, however, it is impossible to imagine major artists repeating this theme. There was, by this time, no settled community with a long tradition of resolving difficulties—nothing like the resolution that we find, for instance, in Sophocles's *Oedipus Rex*, which culminates in *Oedipus at Colonus*, its hero having learned to embrace the larger rhythms of fate and community. Fractures ramified through the whole world that had been colonized by Europe, fractures incident upon the deepest disputes about who we are and how we should live, about the nature of the universe, about the questions of time, of prehistory and history; questions about what the sacred could possibly be, and questions about our ability to participate ritualistically in that sustaining power.

This fracturing only accelerates in the twenty-first century. It is possible, as noted, to speak of the desacralization of Nature that began in seventeenth-century Europe and developed inexorably. Galileo affirmed that the book of Nature is written in mathematical characters. Yet, there was no mathematics that could contain the scope of distinctly human ecstatic activities, so these tended to be regarded by much of the subsequent age as merely subjective and superficial, not fully real (see Fred Kersten, *Galileo and the "Invention" of Opera: A Study in the Phenomenology of Consciousness*). The integrative wisdom of Pythagoras, the Presocratic Greek mathematician, scientist, religious and ethical teacher, musician—previously cited—was apparently lost on Galileo.

The book is not closed on the Romantics, as William Barrett put it (see his *Irrational Man: A Study in Existential Philosophy* and *Time of Need: Forms of Imagination in the Twentieth Century*), nor is it closed on what is to be done with humankind's perhaps insatiable hunger for ecstatic trafficking with sacred energies—with the numinous or the holy—all terms left dangling in the air, dried out and unavailable for very many in the West. Ecstasy still explodes, however, in the widespread and debilitating use of hard drugs, cigarettes, compulsive sex, and alcohol.

We are not at home in the traditional ways—ways that gain their meaning from opposition to the not-at-home or the foreign. I mean the ways that the traditional God and his minions, the angels, gained meaning through opposition to the anti-God, Satan, and his hosts. The composers we confront could manage no clean and clear objectification and splitting of the world into God versus Satan, good versus evil, light versus darkness, us versus them. Polar oppositions and dualisms are too simplistic for them. Still, they probe for primal energies, commitments, involvements; they probe in trackless territories (see, for example, Krishnamurti, "Truth is a Trackless Land" and *Freedom from the Known*).

If time as we live it is measured by the momentousness of change, then the stretch of time from 1800 to 1900—from early and middle Beethoven to Arnold Schoenberg—exhibits as much change as can be found in recorded history. As noted, we live now in ever-accelerating change, as technology, at crucial times the intimate companion of science, easily jumps out on its own, sprouting everywhere faster than weeds, becoming our destiny, it seems.

Over approximately the last three hundred years, we have become habituated to tonal music. For all intents and purposes, it *is* music for most people. I mean the scales that we were taught in school: do, re, me, fa, so, la, ti, and *do*, and the notes that follow again from this *do*. Simplifying now, different "keys" locate their centers on different notes, and create a home for themselves; for example, the key of C is quite different from C-sharp. All kinds of tensions, discords, concords can be found within the chords sounded in each key, and music can sometimes drift or jump into related or distant keys. But we are either at home in the home key or know what would count as finding our way back to it, just as any discord within a home key presents itself as that which is in principle resolvable.

Consider the body's repeated acts of orientation. An instant's orientation must happen when we awaken after each sleep; so quickly does it happen that we probably don't notice it (unless something is very wrong). Successful walking is repeatedly and rhythmically arrested falling. Ears must be especially good at orienting and balancing—why otherwise are they both hearing and balancing organs? We can see only what we are looking at directly in front of us, and we can see directly only surfaces (I postpone dealing with Native American dilation of our experiencing, and with what trackers of animals and birds call "splatter vision"), but we hear what is sounding all around us all at once, and we often can hear into the interiors of things—things that sound on their own or are sounded by other things (see Nietzsche in *Twilight of the Idols*, "Doing Philosophy with a Hammer," that is, tapping things to see if they are hollow—at least that is one of the clear meanings).

In this context, tonal music has been integral to how we have lived, moved, and had our being. It is integral to how we have learned to stand up, walk, reach out, lie down, dance, fight, climb, embrace. It is deeply ingredient in how we have come to locate, orient, balance, and comport ourselves. With its expectation of resolution and well functioning, tonal music has caught on mightily and become integral to our being at home in the world—insofar as we are so. It provides us with a habitual way of handling the much-at-once, of guiding and stabilizing ourselves within its sometimes-shocking turbulences, or of narcotizing ourselves.

But a curious and momentous thing happens with certain composers and musicians in the latter years of the nineteenth century on into the twentieth and twenty-first centuries. They ask: Is tonal music—replete with its returns and resolutions—*true?* Once we think about it, the question is not as outrageous as it may at first sound. How much at home in the world are we? *Are* we balanced and centered? If disrupted, can we find our way home? With vast subjugations and enslavements of peoples; with cruelties, insanities, inanities beyond reckoning; with wars of extermination, genocide? Or beyond this, on its other side, the sheathed-in-India-rubber feeling (James), the terrible boredom, trance, anaesthetization, sleepwalking?

W. B. Yeats intones in "The Second Coming":

> Turning and turning in the widening gyre
> The falcon cannot hear the falconer;
> Things fall apart; the centre cannot hold;
> Mere anarchy is loosed upon the world . . .

It is as if some of the composers we are about to confront in the very early years of the twentieth century were gifted with prescience and prophecy, visitations in their whole bodies, through subtle and not-so-subtle vibrations, from matters gestating, and beyond what they could possibly *say*. It is as if they sensed kinesthetically and aurally the insanities of the upcoming world wars and the probabilities of gas, germ, and atomic warfare. Into this poisonous mix we should also throw, I believe, the trance of technologies, as well as rampaging compulsions and addictions of all kinds. These are dreadful short-circuitings of the regenerative rhythms of Nature, also of course of our own bodies formed in Nature. The composers we will deal with sensed that mere moments—the momentary—would take on a life of their own, and all sense of the overarchingly eventual, as well as the enduringly consummatory, the sacred, would be lost.

Already in Bruckner we find a shying away from the husky dynamisms of the early and middle Beethoven—that is, from what can be called Beethoven's humanist drive for ever-more progress, freedom, and control—whatever exactly all that means. I suggested cautiously that we can read Bruckner's music as a kind of Nature mysticism. Then later, in Mahler, we get Nature again, but also ambiguity, groping, and anxiety. Tchaikovsky's last symphony, particularly its last movement, should also be mentioned—also Nielsen's two "lasts."

What about Beethoven's *Great Fugue*? This music is overwhelming because it taps into the deep structure of the vital self. We experience a godlike power ministering to us and in us. In being a concerted and ever-compounding activity, the fugue empowers our self's ever-compounding creation and recreation of itself: its retention of the past moment, and of what that moment itself retained, and through that further and further back. Also its projection of what it is about to do and be, and where that will take it—the body-self's weaving and reweaving of its being through time and situations as one is followed by another. And not to be forgotten—the fugue's driving exertions consummate themselves in ethereal restings and refreshments—the quiet retrievals of our primal being in ever-regenerative Nature: timely exertion, timely rest, and on and on.

But great as it is, Beethoven's *Great Fugue* is still tonal, and subject to whatever limitations lie within that form of human creation. At least it might clue us in to the self's travails in constituting itself in an ever-driven modern world not congenial to the self's vital creation and recreation of itself. William Barrett writes of an atonal world, one in which changes occur so disruptively that the frameworks developed by humankind over millennia to evaluate matters, to guide and succor itself, fall to pieces (William Barrett, *The Illusion of Technique: A Search for Meaning in a Technological Civilization*). If the meaning of anything is a matter of what we can expect from it for our experience and conduct, and if we cannot count on that actually to happen, at least usually, we don't know what we are doing when we try to project a future. We must doubt our very selves, our continuity, our own reality through time.

In his maturity, Arnold Schoenberg struggled to find himself at home by composing the sounds of a world in which we do not feel at home, are dis-located—an atonal world. That is, he would radically and precariously *make* himself at home, would radically *locate* dislocation. He arrived at this music from a background and a sensibility that is utterly romantic. The somewhat early *Transfigured Night* (op. 4, 1899) is still tonal, though it shifts abruptly from key to key. His composition derives from a poem that, in his own words, is a "highly poetic presentation of the emotions aroused by the beauty of Nature" (program notes, *Verklärte Nacht*, Testament). We encounter a figure reminiscent of Jesus, one who is aroused by the beauties of Nature to create moral beauty. He and a woman walk in a moonlit forest. The woman is carrying a child fathered by a man she does not love. She confesses this to the man with whom she walks and whom she loves. He replies that the love he bears for her will "transfigure your child" so as to become "my own." There is a leap here in self-constitution. Could this sort of thing actually happen, could this generosity and immolation of ego stick, beyond a few moments of high feeling in a moonlit forest? What is there to support the feeling? Schoenberg struggled ever more heatedly with such questions. Can there be a *simul* in that *multis*?

By 1907, with the completion of *Erwartung*, his atonality is in full swing. There is no home key, gone are its reliable chords and their leading rhythms and melodies—no resolutions. This is a world-experienced in which characters cannot balance or orient themselves. All poise is lost. Moments do not hang together for them in any easily intelligible sequence or pattern. It was one-time medical student Arthur Schopenhauer who thought that only music directly conveys the incessant will to live, that which we share with other animals, but this will is typically concealed in us by fine networks of words and pretty appearances. Schoenberg in his music would strip away all fraudulent balance and cohesion. He writes:

> It is impossible for a person to feel only one thing at a time. People feel thousands of things at once. And these thousands of things can no more be summed up than apples and pears. They diverge. And this variety, this multiplicity, this lack of logic that our feelings reveal, this lack of logic demonstrated by the associations revealed by a rising wave of blood or by some physical or nervous reaction—it is this that I should like to have in my music. (Quoted in program notes by Corinna Hesse, *The Romantic Music of Schoenberg*, Telarc)

In *Erwartung*, the world is experienced in hysteria. A woman seeks her lover, and again we are asked to imagine events in a moonlit forest. No clear lines divide shadow from substance, sleep from waking, fact from fantasy, now from then. The ever-compounding fugue-like activity of body-self's constitution of itself through time unravels. The woman does seem to find her lover, but he is dead. The apparent ability of Greek theater to correlate human and animal within a world intelligible to a settled community—what Nietzsche praised so highly—is glaring in its absence. We face instead the reality of hysteria and abandonment for both group and individual. Of course, Schoenberg is *composing* this, not simply experiencing it. I say it again: In his music he is trying to locate our dislocations.

We can describe more concretely and precisely how the woman's grip on reality loosens and fails. She is startled by this and that. What she thinks might happen usually does not. The woman's anticipations are wayward; they don't weave into what actually happens. As suggested before, if the meaning of anything is a matter of what we can expect from it for our experience and conduct, and if we cannot assuredly count on that to happen typically, we don't know what we're doing or who we are when we project a future. More than that, such momentary, failed anticipations pass in the stream of time, and since they have led nowhere, they cannot cohere either with the moments they have superseded or the ones that will supersede them. Projection and retention fail. Identity of self through time flakes away. The failure of the notes to cohere in recognizable tones, chords, intervals, resolutions, keys is essential to the mind and message of the music. This could not have happened with the *Great Fugue*. There, projections or protentions of a future became in time retentions that retained what protentions previous to them had themselves retained, and this repeats, as if a cable of threads were being spun through time. Yet, as I said, Schoenberg is doing his best to *compose* this, and his is a quite remarkable talent!

In a great act of prescience in which the mind of music speaks to our time, Schoenberg creates his three-act opera *Moses und Aron* (circa 1932). Its atonal sounds running independently of one another convey a people who are lost in every conceivable sense of that word. They are not only lost in the trackless Sinai desert for forty years, two generations, but they have lost their bearings in their religious traditions of living. I mean their deeply habituated modes of arising, gaining their balance, walking directedly, dealing with their everyday needs and with each other. These overarching coherences and guidances had been gained in their worship of God, Jehovah. This was now lost. Desperate for a replacement, they ask Moses's brother Aaron to forge and fashion a fertility-figure idol, a young bull calf, out of precious metal. They dance and cavort, they rut, in a pagan Dionysian revel around it; Schoenberg's music conveys this perfectly. But this is not the tradition in which Moses, the leader, wants to plant and replant them. When he returns from his encounter with the Lord on Mount Sinai, he rebukes them. Schoenberg does not follow the biblical story at this point, for he believes that Aaron is let off too lightly in its account. He has Moses put Aaron into chains. Repentant, Aaron is released only to fall dead.

What is an idol? Why is it false? What can possibly be the connection between *any* sign or symbol we fashion and the creative ground of the universe, the *mysterium tremendum*, the Holy, the Sacred? Schoenberg spills us out into the trackless wastes of the secularized, commercialized, technologized, and "entertained" twentieth and twenty-first centuries in which the old hunger for this Power has nevertheless not withered away. It just thrashes about, wayward. The biblical story goes that the lost Hebrews were guided by a pillar of fire by night and a column of white cloud by day. Moses wonders if even these might be diabolical snares meant to deceive them, idols, so long do his and his people's disorientation and despair persist. In this opera, Aaron sings and dances, as does the chorus of the children of Israel; Moses only speaks the Word, though musically (*Sprechstimme*). At the end of the opera—a very strange and revealing one—Moses drops to his knees. What is he to do? Foreseeing our own times, Moses-Schoenberg advises the Israelites to stay in the wilderness, in Nature, for if they join the group of nations there can only be trouble.

We do sense that heroic arias would ring false at this point. Even great previous tonal renderings of Satan (by Berlioz, Liszt, or the earlier Arrigo Boito) have projected him as a being "out there," distinguished from ourselves. We now see that this was naive, for Satan is actually manifest as satanic impulses that occur in our own troubled experiencing of the world: satanic impulses that knot, tear, contort, unravel us as we thrash about frightened or enraged, our identity falling apart and flaking away through time. Boito, for example, labored for decades on an opera in which the diabolical is incorporated into human life itself: *Nerone,* or *Nero* (see the version conducted by Gianandrea Gavazzeni; there is also a good, though very expensive, version with Eve Queler). Aware of the great difficulties, he could never bring himself to complete and stage it, though it does exist in a somewhat reconstructed state. The fourth and last act opens, brutally rhythmical: a kind of rapid stalking sound, but impossibly rapid and peg-legged, uncanny. It conveys the more than human, which is also less than human: that is, the demonic. It raises the hair on the back of the neck.

Schoenberg's Moses is a model self, yet even he must live in the world as it is. His protentions or anticipations don't cohere with the huge corporate individual, the "family of nations." His expectations are not coherently and steadily magnetized by the prospect of Israel at home in this overarching family. Even his identity through time is shaken as he falls to his knees. We as well may shudder when we confront our current reality: corporate individuals—Judaism, Christianity, Islam, our own neoconservative ideologues—armed to the teeth, steeled and fixated in a kind of trance, trying to out-stare each other, set on collision courses.

A bit after Schoenberg's freely atonal period, he developed the so-called serial technique of composition. A row of twelve tones, a tone row, was laid down initially. The rule was: No tone was to be used again until all the others had been used. It's as if he were trying deliberately to undermine our most natural adjustments, rhythms, balancings, spontaneities, connections, harmonies, repetitions. But the rationale is clear. He doesn't trust these in the current state of development of the human race. They aren't *true.* Is he observing arrested development in the race? He may be trying to give us shock therapy. Schoenberg seems to sense that we must become *radically* creative, that we must find ways of coping with, adjusting to, the strangest new circumstances. He struggles to find a new level of continuity and identity. New ways of composing something like a fugue that can empower us, that can re-locate us. I think that he is trying to rediscover the sacred, to find a nearly lost strand and somehow interweave it in our lives (see George Rochberg, *The Aesthetics of Survival: A Composer's View of Twentieth-Century Music*).

Let us turn briefly to two of Schoenberg's students, Alban Berg and Anton Webern. As with the master, Webern is much concerned with Nature and some sort of regenerativity (in this regard, I might have dwelt on Schoenberg's *Pierrot Lunaire,* or *Pierrot of the Moon*). In Webern's Cantata no. 1 (for soprano, choir, and orchestra, op. 29) his atonal technique aims to shake us loose from encrusted ways of taking Nature for granted. Might we regain a sense of its sacred, magnetizing, and supportive power? For example, what if we could retreat to the wilderness for a while and reset our calendars according to the moon's cycles, as was true for our earliest ancestors? Mightn't this break up encrusted "jetlagged" habits and facilitate a reacquaintance with ourselves, our bodies and surround, so that we would gain recuperative experience, as Gabriel Marcel called it? The gradual spading up and turning over of the soil, that tilling of body-self that occurs, breaking up bad trance? For me, at least, when I attend closely, Webern's cantata sometimes succeeds in its regenerative work. Two stanzas in translation:

> The lightning spark of life flashed
> down from the Word-giving cloud.
> Thunder, the heartbeat, follows after
> and then dies away in peace.
>
> Little maple-seed wings floating in the wind:
> You must soon fall to the darkness of earth

> But you will rise up again to the sky,
> to all the fragrance of the springtime;
> you will climb from your roots to bright heaven
> and soon will also take root in the sky.
> And then you will again send out your little wings,
> which already carry in themselves your whole
> silent life, articulate form.
>
> (Nonesuch LP, notes by Eric Salzman)

There is a strong feeling here for the regenerativity of Nature, but also evident, I think, is a mentalistic prejudice in favor of upwardness and light over darkness and earthiness. Still, the words are worthy of citation because the emphasis on regenerativity continues a strand in Schoenberg's work that should be taken seriously. Webern's clipped, minimalist style of composition prompts the regenerativity theme to jump out at us.

With the other of Schoenberg's chief students, Alban Berg, it is quite a different matter. Typically, if Nature is present in his music's mind, it is only as a backdrop to our alienation from her. Berg's famous first opera *Wozzeck,* written between 1914 and 1922, derives from Georg Büchner's nineteenth-century play. It concerns a frantic and demented soldier who is exploited by every sector of society. To say that he is objectified and treated as a mere thing to be examined and used would be gross understatement. Nothing is sacred—not even close to it—no persons, nothing. So extreme is the situation, and so accented and underlined by Berg's atonal music, that we might regard his opera as a kind of thought-experiment. Can we live a life totally devoid of the sacred? Without the magnetizing and directive power of the sacred, can our lives hold together day by day, with any meaning, direction, vitality? Büchner's and Berg's answer, as I hear it, is negative.

The soldier commits a murder and throws his bloody knife into a lake on a moonlit night. As just mentioned, Nature is present only as a backdrop for human alienation from her. Moreover, he has killed a woman. This, and the fact that menstrual cycles of women have become coordinated with the cycles of the moon over countless millennia—and of course are regenerative, essential to the human race's survival—cannot help but figure in our experience of this pivotal opera. The very sources of life are under attack, although Berg's work can *perhaps* also be heard as a lament over this fact.

In Berg's interesting violin concerto (1935), we hear strains from a Bach church cantata *Ich habe genug* (BWV 82)—which can be translated "I have enough" or "I've had enough." "Release me from my shackles," it sings. We might find ourselves singing along with it. If Berg is not merely lamenting our lack of connection to regenerative rhythms, perhaps like his teacher who could work with the twelve-tone limitations as symbolic restriction, he is suggesting that even in these times with limited resources for regeneration, if we can unshackle ourselves, we can still be re-creative with these limited resources?

It would be an oversight to leave twentieth-century attempts to come to grips with music in relation to the deep structure of self without alluding to Sergei Prokofiev and Dmitri Shostakovich (I might also have considered at length the American composer Charles Ives). Although most of this music is tonal, it strains at the leash. Prokofiev's piano sonatas are *possessed*—angelically or demonically? The question fails to gain purchase, which is informative. Traditional, simplistic, binary oppositions and facile dualisms no longer hold in the trackless wastes of twentieth-century experience. This music certainly conveys *something*. Perhaps we can say it reveals ecstatic life that has burst out of traditional frameworks of composition, performance, evaluation. It is music's mind trying to find patterns of anticipation and recall, of guidance and balance, within a chaos of energy: a baffling, often overwhelming much-at-once. Prokofiev's music sometimes succeeds brilliantly.

Consider his 1920s opera in five acts *L'Ange de Feu*, or *The Fiery Angel* (op. 37), which serves a revelatory function for the age. Can we make sense of our animality-humanity? Assuming that we cannot live vitally without some sense of the sacred, can we spiritualize, so to speak, our sexuality? Can we find something like the old Greek satyr-icons in sight, sound, tactility, proprioception and movement, and perhaps olfaction? How do we cycle and gravitate around icons and hold our lives together with focus today? (Also consider Robert Mapplethorpe's photographic—ritualistic?—attempts to aestheticize the penis.) Prokofiev's opera concerns a woman with a quest. She seeks a visitation from an angel. She finds an angel, but it is a fiery one: The angel burns with a dazzling sexual aura. She craves the angel. It is not clear that she ever consummates her passion, nor is it clear what—in our imagination—could count as her doing so. Her raving yearnings prompt the townspeople to arrest her as a witch. "So you want to burn, huh?" Prokofiev finds music to convey contemporary secular humanity's excruciating difficulty in pulling itself together, in integrating its animality with its spirituality. In conveying this, Prokofiev is pulling something important together and articulating it. We are articulated as very like nonhuman animals, and also as very different. We are articulated as paradoxical.

Similar themes and questions emerge with Shostakovich's output. In the 1920s he leapt into world prominence at age nineteen with his exciting First Symphony (Symphony no. 1 in F Minor, op. 10). A prodigy, nevertheless he continued to grow. At about age thirty he produced an opera in four acts, *Lady Macbeth of Mtsensk* (op. 29). This Lady Macbeth is a creature of unbridled, even violent, sexual promiscuity. The opera caused a sensation. When the dictator Joseph Stalin attended its performance, he walked out scandalized—and probably frightened. For societies have always found sexuality the most difficult of human energies to channel, to keep within some bounds. The complex Greek model can be consulted. For Stalin's avowedly secular—or outright atheistic—regime, the challenge presented by Shostakovich's opera was greatly disturbing. Communist ideology inspired the minions, the apparatchiks, to functionalize sex. Free love was advocated, but mainly as a biological need and as a necessity for perpetuating the race and the Communist Party. Its potentially explosive emotional or spiritual charge was to be systematically defused; all connection to "selfish" religious trance states or conversion experiences were to be eliminated. Stalin's inverted Puritanism produced a perfect horror of a society.

Lady Macbeth of Mtsensk was savagely attacked in the state-controlled press, which forced its cancelation. The Stalinist reign of terror had already begun. Contemporaneously with composing his opera, Shostakovich was writing a fourth symphony. In rehearsal at Leningrad (later St. Petersburg), the orchestra and conductor were so apprehensive about performing that Shostakovich withdrew it. It was not performed for twenty-five years—which placed this after the dictator's death. A fifth symphony was composed and was presented with a kind of confession from the composer: "A Soviet musician's response to just criticism." The

Fifth Symphony (Symphony no. 5 in D Minor, op. 47) is not without quality, though quite conventional in every way. Only a genius composer could have contrived it: perhaps the most brilliant potboiler ever set down in notes?

Though appearing within the radiation zone of Mahler (and I think Bruckner), the Fourth Symphony (Symphony no. 4 in C Minor, op. 43) is a great pioneering work of art, groundbreaking, a contribution to tilling the soil of the contemporary human race. It is lengthy, but comprises only three movements, with each movement featuring a tremendous eruption, a brutal crescendo. These increase in force, movement by movement, and culminate in the last. The symphony ends very quietly, with single notes on a harp, suggesting the ticking of a clock. Is time running out for us? The silence that follows is only distantly reminiscent of Bruckner.

Each time these eruptions appear they are eerily foreshadowed—anticipated—without telegraphing the punch. They appear with the power of the *mysterium tremendum*, emerging suddenly from a depth of our being-in-the-world that very probably could not have been predicted, so ambiguous and prelinguistic, so uncontainable is it. I doubt whether Shostakovich would have called them eruptions of the sacred, but given his precarious situation, his demurring would be understandable. I read them as eruptions of the creative powers of the universe. The sacred powers of the *mysterium tremendum* are inherently ambivalent, as already noted; the attraction of adoration is laced with the repulsion of dread. Granted, though, the eruptions in the Fourth Symphony are more heavily weighted on the side of dread.

Indubitably, this symphony pertains to the deep structure of the body-self. We anticipate in some way—perhaps suddenly—an impending future, and more often than not it does occur. The more momentous it turns out to be, the more vividly it is retained, and retained as well is all that comes in the retention's wake. The composer's repeated eruptions reverberate disturbingly down the dark corridors of our experience. Thus the whole work sets our human selves reverberating; It reiterates and recapitulates that fugue-like, self-compounding activity that constitutes who we are. We fugal beings hear the crescendo of the second movement along with that of the retained first movement, then the crescendo of the third movement along with the eruptions of the second and first movements. First in the silence, then in the quiet ticking of the closing measures, the whole symphony soaks through us, buoys and strangely energizes us. We have been met. The music is *true to us*. Though strained greatly, there is a *simul in multis* structuring the symphony. As creatures that are held together fugally, we participate ecstatically in the musical work of art; it responds to our needs for composure in a menacing world (see recorded versions conducted by André Previn and Simon Rattle).

A connection to Bruckner is not completely farfetched. Each eruption is a wave that breaks and rushes up on the shore, then recedes into the belly of the water to recollect itself. The gigantic third and final wave breaks and rushes high up on the shore, then recedes deep into the belly of the water, there to re-collect itself for an indefinite number of further waves—or so we probably anticipate (though I'm not sure). This presents itself as a power beyond reckoning. It is not perfectly clear that we experience in Shostakovich a godlike power to help us and to angelically regenerate us as we do in Beethoven's *Great Fugue* or in much of Bruckner. It may be experienced as carrying a demonic tinge, reminding us that we live on the far side of easy, crystal clear, and simple distinctions: sacred/secular, holy/demonic, good/evil, us/them, and so forth. We live in ambivalence, which suggests the ever-present possibility of pitching off-balance, the possibility of the diabolical or the demonic. Some may hear in this symphony the end of time or the end of the world.

One thing is perfectly clear, however: The Fourth Symphony carries ecstasy and power that lies well beyond the power of any "scientific" secular state to control, beyond the power of marketing managers in the West, beyond fundamentalist coteries in any of the established religions. This ecstasy and power feeds and reassures people open to it who are sick of superficial rationalisms, facile dualisms, splashy entertainments, clever and unrelenting propaganda, and salesmanship from every quarter. Can we call it the relentless peppering of our world by the tinhorn heroic? I'll try another metaphor. Perhaps people feel what most cannot articulate: the monstrous, numbing, bony grip of the contemporary much-at-once, oblivious of any future it helps to produce, pressing hard first on one's fears, then on one's self-doubts, one's greeds and lusts, generally on one's flimsy "self-image"—each one of these as points of vulnerability.

After the semidiversion of Shostakovich's Fifth Symphony comes the magnificent Sixth (Symphony no. 6 in B Minor, op. 54): It commences with a vast lamentation, an adagio, that takes up the lion's share of the three-movement work. Lamentation becomes the ruling mood delivered also in the great Shostakovich symphonies that follow the Sixth, that is the Eighth, the Tenth, the Fifteenth: It is the ground-level mood of sadness, grief, last-ditch dealing with what has been lost. In these later works, the crashes, clashes, and eruptions are more topical and episodic than in the Fourth Symphony, not as earthshaking or, as one might say, cosmic. One can wonder if Shostakovich's regenerative power ever fully reaccumulated after suffering the brutal abortions performed by Stalin and his minions in the ministry of arts and culture. Called before a tribunal of "music critics" were the composers Shostakovich, Prokofiev, and Nikolai Myaskovsky. There, in a show of great courage and pluck, Prokofiev is said to have risen, turned his back to the tribunal, and said in a voice loud enough to be heard in the room, "What do they know about music?"

The great adagio symphonies, which Shostakovich calls his "tombstones," typically contain one or more short, fast movements. These are rollicking and humorous, or grotesque, sarcastic, defiant thumbings of the nose at all conceivable proprieties and pieties. They perform much the same function as did the satyr play, the sex farce that followed the trilogy of tragedies in Greek theater, offering relief from tragedy so that life becomes bearable, so it can go on. They are eruptions out of what can too easily become crushing, crashing, entranced grief—or ghastly boredom. I think that the great music of our time conveys the truth of our condition in a way that nothing else does or can.

As Bruckner was ahead of his students, so the great composers who followed him were ahead of the age. Schoenberg's Moses anticipated the terrible problems of "the family of nations" in the twentieth and twenty-first centuries, and advised the children of Israel to remain in the wilderness. We are inherently social creatures who must bond in groups, but our groups—obsessed with defining themselves as against other groups—threaten to clash and incinerate the planet, threaten to create pan-genocide. The philosopher Karl Jaspers speaks of the New Fact: that for the first time in our history we have the means to destroy life as we know it on this planet. The New Fact combines with old ones: humanity's too often sheep-like foolishness, fear, fickleness, irritable anger. We can create havoc on an astronomical scale that can't really be grasped.

In his very last works Shostakovich quotes passages from Beethoven, Rossini, Wagner, and creates heart-gripping nostalgia. The message we hear in Shostakovich's last nostalgic constructions and quotations: There is no going back, we must go on—a sensibility Shostakovich shares with Samuel Beckett. This man's nation, the corporate body of which he was a part, was headed by a monster. In his memoir, *Testimony: The Memoirs of Dmitri Shostakovich*, he recounts how after one of his pieces was performed he would sometimes be invited for a private chat with Stalin. He did not know whether he would walk back out the door a free man. But he endured the anxiety and kept on composing.

Sacred energies are those that are unconditionally valuable because they bind us ecstatically into the vast experienced world in which we are engulfed. They aren't valuable simply as means to something else that is valuable; they are valuable in and of themselves, intrinsically. Fusing us into the generative and regenerative powers of the world and forming our very core—if we can call it that—they sting our interest and command our devotion. Boredom is impossible. Trading sacred energies for something else is monstrously stupid. We can say that it amounts to viciousness toward oneself, as well as toward others, for whom one cannot help but be a role model.

The current and the preceding few centuries are ones of disruption, alienation, uprootedness—particularly of dis-location. John Dewey states concisely, "The world seems mad in preoccupation with what is specific, particular, disconnected" (*Experience and Nature*, 295). Today sacred energies crop out here and there, but seldom in ways that strengthen us—that bind us into the world-whole and sustain a life day after day, generation after generation. Unless I am very wrong, our deepest need is to ecstatically feel *real*, to feel ourselves to be vital and effective organs in the organic whole of the world. Since a sacrament is that activity that bonds us within the sacred energies of the world, we can say that our ultimate need in a dominantly secularized world is to find a new order of sacraments.

We might find a clue to this new order of sacraments in the anecdote told by Conger Beasley Jr. He recounts accompanying an official of the

Alaska Department of Fish and Game. The goal was to shoot four seals so that biologists could analyze blood and tissue samples for toxins, trace minerals, and parasites. Revolted, Beasley groped for some redeeming qualities in the experience. After a seal is shot, a cloud of its blood boils up around it in the icy water. The redeeming feature is there: For the first time he realized viscerally his consanguinity with seals. He was bonded to a fellow mammal. As they opened up its abdomen, Beasley noted, "I developed an identification with it that carried far beyond mere scientific inquiry. . . . The abdomen of an adult harbor seal is approximately the size of an adult human male's. Each time I reached into the tangled viscera, I felt as if I were reaching for something deep inside myself. As I picked through the sticky folds of the seal's heart, collecting worms, I felt my own heart sputter and knock." As they extirpated the seal's vital organs, Beasley realized viscerally that "the physical body contains functional properties, the proper acknowledgement of which transforms them into a fresh order of sacraments." Coiled intestines intertwine and resonate with the coiled intestines of all animate things. In the recoiling intake of air, in the gasp of awe induced involuntarily in our bodies, we partake of the wilderness *mana* energies we share with all animals. In the intake of breath, we let them into our being. The sacrament is the involuntary acknowledgment of our kinship and common preciousness and power—one that resonates, nevertheless, through our voluntary consciousness and career. It is sacrifice of ego: the acknowledgement of all we do not know and cannot control, upon which we depend. It names the sacred (Conger Beasley Jr., "In Animals We Find Ourselves"; a version of this paragraph appears in Wilshire, *The Primal Roots of American Philosophy*, 58–59).

Is my clue correct that our bodies have a regenerative or sacramental tie to the much-at-once? Are sacred energies those that circulate through all beings—including ourselves—in the much-at-once? To try to suppress these energies is therefore to be diabolical or demonic. Taking this further: Essential to us, and to our vitality, is that we are mineral beings as well as living things—organisms that use signs and symbols widely, with wild energy—but beings that can encounter obdurate matter and rebound in greed, fear, destructiveness, and self-deception. Through scientific reasoning and experiment the so-called strong force that holds the positively charged protons together in the nucleus of atoms has been discovered by us, we humans. Then—of all things!—methods for releasing this force were also discovered, and bombs a thousand times more powerful than those that destroyed whole cities in Japan were created. Only astronomical numbers begin to comprehend this power. The whole significance of it eludes us.

Very probably, we are too vulnerable, defective, limited, and unstable to be entrusted with the unleashing of what amounts to divine power. But our ecstatic thrust propels us to try to understand the welters of things that are happening. To attempt to live without considerable ecstasy is suicidal. Addictions of all sorts are short-circuitings of circular power returning into itself—traumas—as Emerson and also Nietzsche discerned quite some time ago (see Wilshire, *Wild Hunger: The Primal Roots of Modern Addiction*). And because we need to be bonded into the inorganic world as well, I proceed in Segment 4 to look for a new order of sacraments in the world of mineral beings. My hope is that if we can learn to be more at home in the world and with ourselves—with the more-than-human world—and to be less fearful, we might gain the chance to live sanely and well. We might lose the frightened desire to play God.

SEGMENT FOUR

BREAKING THE TRANCE OF MENTALISM

In a cleft that's christened Alt
Under broken stone I halt
At the bottom of a pit
That broad noon has never lit,
And shout a secret to the stone.

—W. B. Yeats (from "Man and the Echo")

We can bond ecstatically not only with birds and fellow animals—particularly mammals—but also with mineral beings such as stones, whether considered "precious" or not. When modern science emerged in the seventeenth century, it was in a mechanistic version: The ruling metaphor for grasping the material universe or Nature was the machine. A machine is composed of neatly separable parts. Where the tooth of a driver gear impinges the tooth of a driven gear, for example, is a precisely demarcated area of material: We know just where the first gear stops and the second begins. It is not surprising that the reality of gears is considered to lie within the boundaries of each of their surfaces, and is equally unsurprisingly that matter so understood was considered "dead." Matter stayed neatly where it was put and could neither ultimately be created nor destroyed by us, although it seemed as if it could be.

In the ensuing centuries, under the impact of evolving systems of physics and biology, the idea of matter evolved radically. It was conceived as one manifestation of a more fundamental reality: energy. Whatever this is in precise terms, it is not neatly and finally contained within the surfaces of gross objects; under certain conditions it can flow, jump, spread amazingly rapidly, explode, at times with stupefying power. Matter can be destroyed, with the resultant release of tremendous amounts of energy. Matter as congealed energy is now best understood not mechanically but organismically, within alterable networks of interdependency, relativity, and flow. When we speak of the matter of a functioning human organism, say, we might speak of it as the miracle of matter.

As noted already, we exist with other things intercorporeally and interfusingly. Dionysus is no longer a fantasy but a greatly revealing metaphor for the contagiousness of reality. What happens when we experiment with the atomic structure of a heavy mineral such as uranium? There's no telling in advance, yet we found that it disastrously changed who we are. Employing our powers of scientific curiosity and investigation and our advanced technologies, we learned about the structure of its nucleus. Then we learned how to "split" it and release the stupefying energy of the powerful force that holds it together. Ironically, we have so "successfully" created a weapon that it is too powerful to use, though it may be used against us. Clearly, there is vastly more that we must learn about *ourselves*—our fears, emotions, motives, trances—and science as we know it is necessary but not sufficient to achieve this knowledge (for science, to be successful, must limit its vocabulary and methods, must rule out investigation of some of the things that would have destructive impacts upon us, since we realize we are not at an impervious remove from them). How do we contend with what amounts to sacred power, sacred energy? Without a linkage to keen new insight, to commonsense and morality, the sacred runs wild in the worst sense. This is what I struggle with in this book.

I propose to look more closely at the evolving idea of matter, particularly at how the seventeenth-century mechanistic physicist René Descartes formulated a seminal account of the mental or spiritual that does not reveal ourselves to ourselves; it obscures us instead. For perversely enough, he smuggled into his account of the "mental" or "nonphysical" a somewhat disguised simulacrum of his mechanistic idea of matter—and that as "dead," inert and safely contained. Descartes does not look and listen to what actually happens when we live, know, and perceive (or misperceive) in the world, our actual awareness and minding. He reifies a mere phrase, "the mind," and his idea of Nature is "subnatural."

One of the great wrong turns in the history of thought—perhaps the greatest—was taken, I believe, in the seventeenth century by this audacious scientist, philosopher, soldier, and mathematician. Prior to Descartes, a stable assumption (or category of thought) had pretty well dominated: That along with the being or reality of actual things, substances and their attributes, as well as the being or reality of truth, there is the being or reality of *potentiality.* This point was made long ago by Aristotle, but in light of the huge influence of Descartes, we need to consider it afresh.

Descartes would not accept this old idea. Reality had to be *actuality* in some form: whatever occurs here and now in some point-instant and can be denoted and pinned down some way. If it is physical actuality, it must be characterizable precisely by mathematics and measurement. One of Descartes's great scientific feats was analytic geometry: conceptualizations that linked geometrical shapes to algebraic equations. This brought a major advance in the quantification of matter and Nature, which prepared for North Atlantic industrialization by reducing the world to measurable and manipulable units—what some have called the "disenchantment of the world."

Then, for Descartes, there is mental actuality, an actuality that is nonextended and noninertial, comprising mental simples or "atoms," simple ideas, irreducible mental images, and similar. These occur somehow "in the mind" in some point-instant. They are not precisely characterizable mathematically, but they are real because actual in actual minds here and now. Mind is equated in Descartes's thinking with consciousness, a supposedly personal and private consciousness, which is essentially self-reflexive, self-grasping. Because it holds itself together and in a sense stands all by itself, it is construed by Descartes as a substantial reality, a substance, even though nonphysical. What is "in the mind" or in consciousness in the point-instant? Well, it must be some kind of mental entity—some visual or auditory image or some sensation—and given that it is *in* consciousness, Descartes infers that consciousness must be *aware* of it.

This inference is later hotly contested by Charles Peirce and William James. For these, our thinkers, the whole Cartesian approach is the stupendous and stupefying wrong turn that must be reversed. Descartes's assumptions—his actualism, mentalism, atomism, substantialism—tend to blind us to our own lives as minding organisms caught up dynamically moment to moment in the much-at-once of the experienceable world. Actually, our thinkers discern that Descartes's view is a covert and perverse materialism—a "physics" of the "internal or subjective domain"!

What is the reality of that which immediately appears to us? What appear are not private, mental entities. What appears, rather, is what is the case: that we are organisms along with others awash in the much-at-once of a world that is experienced prereflectively. We cannot begin to allude to what is "private" in our experiencing without presupposing things in the world that are perceived in common with others. It is *that thing* we both see on the table—that dish of asparagus—that perhaps tastes quite different to each. Contra Descartes, abundantly more flows by in our immediate experiencing than we ever become consciously aware of. If reflection and analysis occur, they do so a moment too late, picking up only the crumbs that fall from the feast of the ongoing, world-involved, spontaneous, prereflective life. They screen out as much as they reveal.

Our thinkers maintain that the mechanistic physicist-philosopher Descartes has smuggled into his worldview a reflective analysis of "mental life" in the image of quasi-physical "atoms"—an analysis that forgets itself. The wide world in which we are immediately involved is obscured, and our involvements are likewise obscured, dampened, warped. Our thinkers perceive the febrile and debilitating advent of scientism: that which is a counterfeit of science. James proposes that the primal reality of what we may call mental life is really *sciousness*—his neologism. It is not *con-sciousness,* not awareness of awareness, for we are primally aware *pre*reflectively of many of the world's actualities and potentialities. We are open, porous, vulnerable, aswim in immediate involvements in a shared world. Moreover, as porous organisms adapting as best we can to things around and in us, we know more than we *know* that we know—much more than we can reflect on and acknowledge, and far more than we can say. To miss this point is to be locked out of vital animal life with all its spontaneities, surprises, gains, losses, and sudden openings of this or that horizon.

More is at work on and in us than we can ever fully know. Our moody awarenesses find us surprisingly. In his essay entitled "Nature," Emerson writes of a particular visitation within the much-at-once: "Crossing a bare common, in snow puddles, at twilight, under a clouded sky, without having in my thoughts any occurrence of special good fortune, I have enjoyed a perfect exhilaration. I am glad to the brink of fear" (*Nature and Selected Essays,* 38). Emerson is unexpectedly ecstatically touched by the power of the sacred.

Mind is not a substance but a function, the organism's ways of *minding*, and these are ways of being led around—or misled—as organisms within the dense, throbbing world and all its challenges to navigation (which does not rule out being led by theory, and then perhaps to yet more theory). Most of what we are aware of is not in the acknowledgeable and articulable focus of awareness, but occurs on the margins of awareness and is never articulable verbally, at least not in prose or in mathematics. The margins fade out indefinitely on every side, above, below, and behind, and cannot be precisely marked, but are real as ever-present actualities *and* potentialities of world and world-involvement: the much-at-once.

More important, what is registered in our minding need not be in awareness—in *sciousness* or consciousness—at all (see Dewey, *Experience and Nature*). Most of the time we live in an experienced world that is mainly out of focus; we are often only blurrily aware of it. Our organisms embedded in the moving world simply tend one way or the other, we are moved in some nisus or other, living in one degree or another of *trance.* It is a prereflective attunement, such as varied animals have toward their environment. Take, for example, a skilled and capable driver of a car. In the field of the driver's awareness can be a thousand matters other than driving, and usually safely so, as long as things go smoothly. One is aware of what's happening on the road, but not focally: One is aware on the margins of awareness and in a *trance* state. The chief reason that using a cellphone while driving is dangerous is that it easily distracts us from the nonfocal but essential *trance awareness* of what's going on before and around us. Using the cellphone overoccupies us as minding organisms while we drive.

Hence minding cannot be a matter of having discrete mental states here and now, but of occupying some imprecise area in a continuum of the organism's various sorts of minding, with some degree of sensed potentiality always active, at least in the margins of the evolving fugal developments of our ecstatic lives. Charles Peirce defines *continuum* as that reality that is not "constructible" by thought out of any number or kinds of units. There are no precise, sharp-edged states, boundaries, stages, segments, ultimate monads, or atoms of any sort, but an essentially blurry—yet profoundly real—processual life to be lived.

The danger in referring to the *continuum* of experiencing is to reify and spatialize it, in turn, as a linear extent or stretch of some kind of rarified substance or stuff. As we aware organisms roam through the world—or are shoved or pushed or niggled and teased along—we are remembering, perceiving, anticipating, imagining things. We are moved according to certain hunches, and at the same time suffering, enjoying, regretting, exulting, or whatever—maybe scratching our heads about what is happening. Our experiencing life is as multiplex and variable as the much-at-once that works on us from every side every moment, from within and without. To think that we are duplex or composite beings—constituted by two forms of substance, mental and physical, somehow in tandem—is preposterous. It is the work of a desacralized, driven, pinpointing, vision-dominated worldview.

Friedrich W. J. Schelling, a great and greatly neglected nineteenth-century thinker, asserted that in important art, conscious and unconscious motivations combine in the art's eruptive creation. Consider intense creativity in music, for example: The characteristics with shifting values, voices, and sounds that can be factored out are, at a minimum, loudness, pitch, timbre (brightness of tone), melodic line, tempo, rhythmic variation, and so on. Moreover, consider in addition all the characteristics of the actually or potentially moving, functioning, balancing, listening, attitude-taking human body. Artists and audience are finding new ways of being alive in the world, new insights, communications, discoveries, angles, enjoyments, hunches, premonitions. Whether they can acknowledge them or not, or deal with them well, they are being touched by sacred interfusions and energies.

Intense musical creativity is a kind of trance as delirium, in which more impulses and elements are involved in intersection and fusion than can be picked out, enumerated, calculated, controlled. It is a spontaneously evolving, emotionally moving, self-organizing whole that draws the composer, musicians, ourselves the listeners—and incipient or actual dancers—into itself as if into a vortex. In other words, it is an ecstatic trance-state that can be difficult to break out of. We resent interruptions, hence the "notoriously temperamental composers and musicians." We are brought home to ourselves as the incredibly complex, situated, temporal organisms that we are. We are reminded that dualisms and polar oppositions badly oversimplify and obscure the beings that we are. We should be gripped by the momentous question of our freedom as agents, as selves. No "free will" drops down from the sky as an undeserved gift. We must work and endure and allow certain impulses to happen if we are to be the effective free agents that at times we certainly seem to be.

Freedom requires the willingness and ability to do the valuable thing, or to let it happen: As Emerson would say, the ability at crucial moments to abandon calculation, the attempt to totally control. It is no mere "indeterminacy of the will." The real meaning of freedom is allowing powerfully creative processes to grip, pull, propel, and direct us. A leap of faith in our freedom will be effective when it is triggered by powerfully creative trance or trance-like insights and intuitions—eruptions of construction and creation, perhaps great fugues. There are good trances and bad ones.

Thus we reconsider today the function of the chorus in Greek tragedy. How do we take that half-step back within our ongoing much-at-once and, without losing touch with this evolving circumpressure, enlarge the context in which we evaluate what is happening? If the moment is a veritable delirium of creativity, this half-step back may be impossible.[1] But another moment will come, in which the previous moment resounds—in

1. We might consider the delirium of creativity as the least mechanical of the trances, but the whole polar opposition of "mechanical versus organismic" can be used only with extreme caution. The purposive, potential, end-directedness of human life exists in a myriad of forms and degrees. Thus we might be tempted to say that someone in a hypnotic state acts mechanically. Yet if the hypnotist suggests that hypnotized subjects do something that the persons believe to be dangerous or immoral, they typically will not do it. It is plausible to assume that a sense of potentiality and agency never completely deserts persons even when hypnotized. We are also tempted to imagine that in periods of intense creativity, more ends or goals are active in the creator's much-at-once than can be itemized or controlled. It is like a delirium, a whirlpool that pulls us into itself. Although this suggests an organismic metaphor, it is not nearly as dangerous as the mechanistic metaphor, and in fact it may be greatly helpful.

other words, the fugue-like life of the self is going on, *simul in multis.* In general, the challenge is: How do we as chorus, without losing the moment, move beyond the moment in thought? How do we assess and evaluate as a group what is happening, has happened, or will do so imminently?

A genius in any sort of endeavor—scientific, artistic, religious, political, commercial—is of course extraordinary, but a genius in practical wisdom—in knowing how to live well—is especially extraordinary: Heraclitus, Socrates, Moses, Aristotle, Jesus. Consider just the last two. Aristotle knew that attaining a significant degree of practical wisdom required that, at some pivotal times in each of our developing lives, we have be taken by the hand, perhaps literally, by a wise person. It is *hands-on,* immediate, repetitious, habit-forming, bodily learning. Jesus knew that if one would save one's life, one must lose it. Each of us, to find ourselves, will have to lose ourselves ecstatically in some work or cause that claims us, claims our belief, respect, devotion, intimate involvement.

In Part II of this book I touch on world-historical geniuses in the American mold: Thomas Jefferson, R. W. Emerson, and Charles Peirce, in addition to William James and the Native American Black Elk. What might they tell us about the human condition, what it takes to be a full, alive, whole, ecstatic human being—particularly if we read them as if we were aspiring members of a contemporary chorus? Have we had world-historical geniuses witness for us how to live well, husbanding our potentialities for choice in the everyday world? Who exemplify to us the reality of that truth?

Where are we, here and now? There is the glaring light of publicity, the endless clattering of commercial hype, the arrays of factoids along with pictures of people being blown to bits, say—that's the news. But I want to ask where we stand, each of us, in our own bodily, emotional, moody existence moment to moment. That is, is it well with our *souls* as bodily, cultural, experiencing beings? (I have decided to employ the term "soul" at this particular moment of the book, which will mean *all* that the functioning body can do—not implying that we can know what that all is, nor that we can know when or how sacred energies will touch and move us.) Are we glad to be alive and at home in the world because we believe we contribute something positive to the whole amazing thing, that we have some significance?

As pointed out earlier, vision is the distancing and detaching sense par excellence. If we are fully alive, we will know what Yeats is doing when, in the *darkness*, he has his poetically imagined character *shout* a secret to the *stone*. Something nearer than the nearest is happening, something that possesses our inwardness: Our bodies are material, and they have taken shape over hundreds of thousands of years in deepest interfusion with the elements of the earth, with the molecules of air that circulate through us and in which we breathe, walk, speak, dance, and sing, and with all the various encompassing vibrations and impingements of energy that animate our sense organs as well as the interiors of our bodies. What is the secret kinship that, in the darkness, we shout to the stone?

Well, that we're *real* and impermanent congealings of energy, yet also that we refuse to be rubbed out merely at someone's whim: that our *experiencings* and *feelings*, and what we *might* do, are real and that they matter. Among the great emotions are love, anger, fear, anxiety, trust, hope, reverence, endurance. Love includes self-love and self-respect. Each of the great emotions has its distinctive counterpart in corresponding movements of heart and lungs as they throb in the cage of ribs. The heart beats rapidly in fear, calmly in trust and hope. The lungs expand and contract rapidly in great anger, and deeply and slowly in confident trust. The heart and the lungs reside in the chest, even as the mind of music speaks directly to—and out of—the chest.

When we shout a secret to the stone, do we shout the secret of our solidarity with the stone? Might that shouting be a singing and a resonance with the stone? Does it echo us back to ourselves—back into ourselves? Or is it just an object to be perceived within the restricted context of mineralogy, say, or within an immediate project such as digging a well, an impediment to that? Or is it an object to be gazed at detachedly?

It is no accident that the Greeks located the moral virtues and also the great emotions in the chest (*thumos*). Temperance requires the balance of the whole bodily self, and its center of gravity is the chest: The chest *and* the abdomen as the trunk balance confidently on pelvis and legs. Loyalty is a kind of bridge between temperance and courage. There is a clear intellectual component in both temperance and courage, for as Socrates and Plato pointed out, both virtues require knowledge of what ought to be feared, and what should be most honored. "Unrighteousness . . . runs faster than death," said Socrates (Plato, *Apology*, 64), and is more to be feared. Music arouses the great moral virtues, keeping us balanced and effective; Music can buffer us against hysteria, panic, and alienation, not-at-home-ness. So we believe when we keep enduring and creating despite everything.

To be sure, our chests may have become habitually crumpled because of impossible situations in which we have been placed. Trying to avoid florid outbreaks of flying apart in schizophrenia, we may have descended into it, rolling ourselves up into an armored ball like a sow bug or an armadillo. If so, music will probably come too late; we may only hear it at a distance, "out there," as our eyes are misting over. But music may often confirm and bring us home to the best in ourselves. So despite the many disappointments, frustrations, even traumatizing horrors of life, and the fact that we don't live in a settled community of likeminded people, as citizens of the Greek polis did, music may brace, calm, stay us in our innermost resolve. (Moreover, the likeminded community of fifth-century Greece was no unmixed blessing; only an elite segment of the populace could attend public performances of any kind.) We might grow in resolve even to the point that apparently irresolvable difficulties, frustrations, and conflicts don't unhinge us. Perhaps? Even gritty endurance has its ecstasies, though boredom does not.

It is likely that Yeats's protagonist "at the bottom of a pit," encompassed by a depth that broad noon has never lit, is touching the stone as he shouts his secret to it. More likely still, he is leaning his chest against it. He may shout, "I too am real! Your minerals form my bones that are the scaffolding of my flesh and nerves, and my bony and flexible ribs house my heart, lungs, and other vital organs of the trunk. All through my bones, but particularly right here in my ribcage, I vibrate deeply with the indefinitely various resonances of earth, air, water, and sky." And, to be sure, the brain is an integral part of the body, even though we can have no direct awareness of it (see Appendix B on music and the brain).

Sight can pick out only one thing or one field at a time, though in glancing it can jump quickly from focus to focus. Hearing, by contrast, can pick out—if it will—from every direction at once, and the range of hearing is immense: from exceedingly shrill and high sounds to ones that, as we say, are as low as can be heard. It would be clearer if we said that they are as low as we can *acknowledge* we are hearing. Persons really listening can respond to the much-at-once and—poised—know that that they are doing so. They can be at home on the earth, prepared to move out in any direction if need be, but at ease in the place in which they dwell and are at home.

For there is evidence that when sonic vibrations beneath the level of acknowledgement are generated, people's behavior changes in definite ways. These vibrations might constitute the "bass-note of life," following James's metaphor (James, "Is Life Worth Living?" 32). Native North Americans would put their ears to the earth to detect the presence of herds of bison many miles away. It is doubtful that they could hear acknowledgeable "noise"; they felt the vibrations—the sound, or better the sounding, of the bison herds. Call it a harmony that lies beneath the level of easy verbal acknowledgement.

The man in the pit with his chest to the stone was picking up the bass note of reality: the whole world all around and under him, that vast residual presence of the cosmos as it pervaded his body—the much-at-once. Actually, we are always irradiated by the cosmos, but we are conditioned by our culture from birth to notice only the smallest range of things that occur, even in our immediate environment. But we know, in a fundamental sense, much more than we know that we know. Now, can we integrate this knowledge with what we've been conditioned to acknowledge in our enculturation? Or are we doomed ever to be fragments—though perhaps "functional" ones?

It is striking that in ancient Greek cultures some sibyls, prophets, prophetesses, and shamans spoke with a "belly voice," a hoarse second voice that imparted to hearers more than they could typically access articulately (see E. R. Dodds, *The Greeks and the Irrational*, Chapter 3). Presumably these were the people who "had their ears to the ground." Presumably also, this is a dimension of the secret that the man shouted to the stone in response to whatever it had communicated to him.

The sound of industrial machinery tends to obliterate the rhythms and sounds of human organisms at work or play, and of other animals and birds moving about and sounding in their distinctive ways. Machine sounds obliterate vibrations that irradiate us from every quarter of the world, and that we have probably been taught could not be important even if we could imagine them. The full *mind* of music can be obliterated; one may suspect that it is in the process of being so. Agriculture is now agribusiness, and even yard work at home is attacked by mobile industries of trucks and trailers that carry mowers, clippers, whirring spindles of nylon, oppressive leaf blowers. With protectors clamped over ears, the worker seems to be part of the machinery. Efficiency! Efficiency and obliteration. We are not speaking of merely poetic niceties here.

By a measure of inches and feet, we can be close to human and nonhuman things and at the same time weirdly isolated and alone. But in and through the chest and abdomen we *might* resonate with the sounds and vibrations of living things, indeed of the whole ambient as well as the whole mineral world. We should speak of trunk knowledge. In seeing, we must turn toward what is to be seen. In touching, we must reach out to that thing we intend to touch. In hearing we may cock our ears in the direction from which the sound seems to emanate, but our *whole balancing body*—brain included of course—picks up everything from all around, all at once. The great emotions—and the great moods—reside particularly in the trunk. They form a level of reality deeper than mere sensations or the more superficial emotions: If habitually attended to, this level of reality can enter, center, and balance us ecstatically, and perhaps we can also say, sacramentally. I think we should call this the unconditionally valuable, or the sacred.

Our sense of any distance to be traversed is tied ineluctably to our sense of the time it would take to traverse the space. We imagine: What will happen if we traverse this? What is *there* is what it will be like *then*. With these reflections we probe into a primal experience of space-time, entering into the vastness of our own encountering, experiencing, balancing lives in the world, actual and possible, and also into relativity physics (to be further developed in Segment 7).

But for trunk knowledge, the *here* and *now* is not neatly divided from the *there* and *then*. Time smudges and smears: The past may be a haunting presence that crowds to the side what is happening here and now, and the anticipated future can have an overriding presence. Olfaction likewise resides in the whole body and bridges time instantaneously: In the memory of a smell, the past is relived strangely. The moral virtues can be pumped full of life and sustained: patience, loyalty, resolve, courage, faith. *Simul in multis*: we remain fully ourselves, whole beings, through the very multitude of different factors and capacities that are available, that are ours, interwoven and strung through us.

Before any of us could say "I," we had to know our *call*. The persons who first called us located, sustained, identified us. Those persons' vibratory reality still pervades us, typically. If it was oppressive, we will still feel oppressed. If buoying, liberating, and guiding, we will still feel buoyed, liberated, guided. Those persons—did they make us feel good when we went to bed at night, and good when we got up in the morning? Linear time, as a sequence of moments that are continually annihilated as they pass, is real but is far from the whole story about time, including our own time-spanning, time-connecting, our own buoying or oppressing existence.

Our call, what we have been *named*, is that peculiar sound, that utterly unique music—whether legato and soothing, staccato and harsh, or presto and lilting—that singled us out from everything else in the universe and summoned us into the presence of those who recognize us, who witness concerning us in one way or another. Perhaps this has evolutionary roots in the broader animal world, as attested by scientists' recent discovery that dolphins "call each other by name" through a unique whistle (see Rebecca Morelle, "Dolphins 'Call Each Other by Name,'"). To forget the name of a restaurant at which we are to meet a friend, for example, is nothing like forgetting the friend's name when we meet, for by forgetting that name we have taken a step toward obliterating that person's presence and reality (of course, the friend need not feel diminished by our inattention, negligence, or inadvertent forgetfulness). Our call may come from many others around us, even from ancestors far distant from us, if we manage to open up ecstatically to them. Those others may have cursed our lives, or may have blessed them; when we make even the curses our own, acknowledge and encompass them, we are greater thereby. It is odd to say that to be most vitally real and in touch with ourselves, we need to be in touch with what has cursed us, but I think it is true. I think it has that mode of *being*.

Some psychiatrists and psychologists report that the loss of hearing may be a more grievous loss for the patient than that of sight. This may seem surprising to a culture that has prioritized the importance of seeing over hearing, yet hearing seems to have a unique power to immerse us within the more-than-us. In Michael Chorost's book *Rebuilt: My Journey Back to the Hearing World*, for example, he states, "the sense of hearing immerses you in the world as no other. . . . Hearing constitutes your sense of being *of* the world, in the thick of it. To see is to observe, but to hear is to be enveloped" (9). When he first lost his hearing, Chorost felt at a distance from the world; he imagined that his cochlear implant, which would supply a computer-generated equivalent of what he used to hear, would be like being "reborn into another body." Chorost and others in the deaf community he describes have a rich life in the community and the natural world, but have to find other means to nurture this interconnectedness that the music of the world and the music that we make offers immediately to hearing as a simple gift. Chorost and others remark on the body's flexibility in establishing other means to meanings perceived with one sense, alternatively registering it through others. Yet music makes us aware of the aural presence and its rich immersion that we so easily take for granted.

It is not enough that human beings be real things or objects: We must experience ourselves as *persons* or *selves*, must truly feel this reality. To do so, we must be recognized as such by other real persons or selves. We want the world to recognize what we do and are, what we might do, and we want it to echo back to us what we might *be*. Indeed, we want the world to do more than echo, for it should carry real responses of other persons and things back to us, never perfectly predictable. The world is not simply mechanical but is organismic: Novelty and growth—or decay—really do occur. Well-functioning parts are organs that function for the sake of the whole—not only for the whole organism, but for the whole group. The well-functioning and vibrant whole feeds back into each organ. It is not true that we fully experience the world as an isolated perceiving mechanism, if we need others to coperceive with each of us.

Atonal music had a message to carry: The modern world is one in which many Europeans—and those under the influence of Europe—do not feel at home, do not feel adequately recognized, nor adequately challenged in their possibilities. They do not feel confirmed in their reality, do not feel authorized by authoritative others, and by significant tasks that they themselves might do. This is excruciatingly true if their religious beliefs and commitments are undermined. They are severed from the Trunk of the Tree of the World. Here capitalization helps us grasp what both Emerson and Black Elk tried to convey concerning the weight and moment of the full order of the sacred. We must partake in the energies of the world: circular power ever returning into itself.

The contrast with ancient Greek theater is instructive: The audience during the drama identified with the characters enacted and with the chorus circulating around and behind them. The chorus danced and chanted their race's experience as that had funded itself over an immemorial stretch of time. The past was an authoritative presence and it promised guidance for the future. When the chorus chanted to Oedipus, "'Tis Time, Time, desireless, hath shown thee what thou art" (*Oedipus King of Thebes*, 73), their stamping footfalls and voices pounded in the lesson, and the audience presumably heeded it. They were authorized as the people for whom the message was meant.

It was not only twentieth-century atonal music that conveyed the failure of us moderns to be convincingly authorized in our reality; modern drama from Shakespeare through Büchner to Samuel Beckett conveyed the same. The *absence* of the chanting, dancing chorus in all these arts is perhaps the most significant thing about them. Lacking is the authoritative, time-tested, recallable point of view of a community of beings funding itself over time and flowing, communicating, and guiding in manifold ways. This deep consensus with respect to us—particularly when we are growing up—is essential to our conviction that we are real. Throughout this book, I am trying out the idea that the modern audience should face the challenge of becoming a chorus for itself—even if this is a very tall order.

Hamlet is riddled with doubt, about what to do, and about himself. Though his ghost-father has visited him and ordered the son to avenge him on his murderous brother Claudius, Hamlet's uncle, Hamlet delays. Perhaps the ghost was a deceiving minister set upon him by the devil? Perhaps this, perhaps that . . . Lacking to Hamlet is the force of the blind prophet's shocking disclosure to Oedipus long ago, and the force of the chorus's acceptance of this. Hamlet visits his mother alone, he thinks, in her bedchamber. When he remonstrates with her over submitting to Claudius's blandishments, his passionate rage sweats and breathes heavily; it is not too much to evoke Freud's speculations about half-suppressed incest wishes. Yet it may be more relevant to this book's emphasis on the sense of hearing as an opening to the world that Claudius killed King Hamlet by *pouring poison into his ear.*

There was no halfway suppressed anything in Sophocles's *Oedipus Rex.* When Oedipus the king and Jocasta the queen discover that they have committed incest, they discover simultaneously that they have fouled not only the city, but the universe itself—I mean the creativity of the universe, the primordial fact that parents, procreators, must bring up their children so that the children themselves, in the fullness of time, can become creators in their own right. Jocasta's womb cannot both give birth to her son and receive his "casting of the grain." There is no doubt for the Greeks in attendance: The regenerative rhythms and cycles of the universe have been short-circuited, and people walk about half-alive, if they live at all—unless they pay the price for what they have done, unless they give back to the universe something of what they have wrongly taken. Such matters involve us as collective and not isolated individuals, and once heard together, the world must move on to a new place. The universal law is plain, as both Jesus and Sophocles know: We must reach out ecstatically into what we are *not—simul in multis.* We must die to the old so that we can encompass and nurture what might be, should be, is perhaps about to be. We belong to a universe vastly greater than ourselves, and to experience its power is to experience the sacred.

The very essence of music and dance is time, which carries along all bodily beings inexorably. Depending on total context, frenetic music and dance can be a milking of the possibilities of every passing moment, or a frantic attempt to defy the inexorability of time's measured pacing. Slowly phrased music and dance can be a reveling in the possibilities of acceptance, leisure, sensuous or meditative savoring, or it can be a dragging depression and despair. Thrusting and continuous melodies and rhythms, again depending on total context, can exhibit confidence and competence, or a diabolical fixation on achieving some end, a diabolism revealed through grating, disturbing harmonies and dissonances: time without buoying support and refreshment. For Hamlet, "the time is out of joint," and he is fatally out of tune. He has not been adequately authorized in his being.

Thus Shakespeare's drama discloses one of the clear possibilities—inevitabilities?—of fast-evolving and splintering secularism. We do not feel deeply at home in the whole universe that holds us in its grip—cry, scream, wriggle, and kick as we might. No merely intellectual or wordy knowing will restore us to home or to balance and poise. For many, there is no music that can embody our vital reality through the moments of time. Unlike Yeats's man in the pit, we feel nothing for the stone, except maybe impatience.

Samuel Beckett's *Waiting for Godot* is also soaked with time. The characters' daunting task is to learn to cope with it. Their perplexity is an invisible viscous fluid, like oil, in which they can barely stay upright and cannot hear the call or tread of time. Or, they are profoundly bored, sheathed in the India-rubber feeling. They are depicted outside "on a country road," but unlike persons involved in the Greek theater, they are in a theater house, not really outside, and unlike them they do not feel they belong in a people's history. They do not feel the pervading presence of gods and goddesses, nor do they feel that they belong in any time-honored tradition that assigns them roles and provides them with rules. So out of phase with time are they that they cannot trust their memories. Hence they are not sure of who they are: The fugue that they are, or were, has petered out. If there were music in the play, it would be that of stunned foreboding. But there is no music.

The only way they find to deal with time is through time-killers, putting off and on their boots, tapping on the crowns of their hats (looking for their brains?), entertaining themselves with boring sexual jokes, all repetitions little more than mechanical. They are waiting for some authority, Godot (God?) to tell them what to do and who they are. Enter a man with a whip driving a small person before him. It is Pozzo who is driving Lucky. This little person staggers under the baggage he carries and is totally abject. The two tramps are fascinated. Is Pozzo the long-awaited Godot? The slave driver seats his large bulk and gives an order to Lucky, "Think!" Lucky unleashes a spieling flood of words, a string of mainly unrelated names and bits of information, which, once begun, Pozzo has a hard time stopping. The tramps shout, "Stop! Stop!"

In the second act, slave driver and slave reenter. Lucky is dumb and Pozzo is blind. The tramps ask Pozzo when all this happened. Pozzo, suddenly furious, raves:

> Have you not done tormenting me with your accursed time! It's abominable! When! When! One day, is that not enough for you, one day he went dumb, one day I went blind, one day we'll go deaf, one day we were born, one day we shall die, the same day, the same second, is that not enough for you? (Calmer.) They give birth astride of a grave, the light gleams an instant, then it's night once more. (He jerks the rope.) On!

The two reenter, but it is a return without regeneration, to put it mildly. Pozzo's "On," his frantic way of living at a dead run, sustains a false balance.

It is hard to avoid the conclusion that a mirror has been set before us. Evading the visual metaphor, we might say that we have been invited into a situation with which we resonate in our bones. Yes, we have amassed great stores of facts, but do we really much care? Do we believe in the future and in our ability to make some significant difference in how things turn out? Has chronological time become mere pointless, mechanical repetition, devoid of human meaning? For many people, nothing of *for the sake of which* moves them. Nothing of what they might revere and adore does this. They have been reduced, say, to mere addictive acquisition. As Emerson puts it, we humans are capable of degenerating into mere dried-out fragments, not living organs of the whole organismic world.

Tolstoy thought that the most important knowledge is knowing how to live, and that "that by which we live" is a gushing up from deep sources of human vitality: from our role models—or being ourselves role models for others. What gushes up are sacred, numinous presences or icons of grandeur, visual or sonic, or models of moral beauty or of wise and compassionate actions ingrained in our cycling bodies, our beating hearts, our bones and nervous systems. The Bible speaks of the "bowels" of mercy. The life force can burst up and carry us even through sadness, pity, or grief. Without this buoying and sacred power, life is pointless, empty, and flat. We are profoundly bored. In the next part of the book, I will allude to Schopenhauer on music and its direct conveyance to us of the life force, *Wille*, will.

When all these incidents have passed in *Waiting for Godot*, Beckett's tramps say to each other, "Let's go!" and "Yes, let's go." The stage direction reads: *They do not move*. They haven't really heard each other, hearkened to each other. Their words are mere chaff in the wind. That ends the play. We have witnessed a total loss of ecstasy and power, a total spiritual-physical-moral paralysis, emptiness, collapse, dislocation. But the loss has been conveyed, even ecstatically so, witnessing that sacred energies are not totally defunct.

"Life is so daily," the cleaning lady said. We must live in real time, day after day, not just in the real time it takes to unfold the time of the play's world, or the opera's, or the symphony's. Nevertheless, performance is a fundamentally real aspect of our human lives, and humanity is inconceivable without its arts (Dewey classified the sciences as arts; that is, the arts of making precise predictions). Can we better bridge the arts and our daily lives? Along with this question we raise ones posed earlier: Can we become the chorus for the performances? Can we place them in a context in which the full moment of our perplexities and problems today comes home to us?

For us in the United States, it is our country itself that boils and jostles turbidly around us all the time. It is difficult to take as seriously as we once might have Lincoln's presentation of our nation as the "last best hope" of earth—the living ideal of self-governing, self-respecting, and other-respecting persons that forms a new kind of national group under the sun. Honesty requires us to acknowledge that the United States is too often both fearful and arrogant, the one-time colony that acquired colonizing dreams and programs of its own. Now the dreams are garbed in commercial and military power exclusively—gone is the time when the British pith helmet atop the great white hunter and the many florid badges of French *gloire* made the colonizers more obvious. If we could understand and accept our actual situation here and now, we would feel ourselves to be more real, more authorized, more centered and poised. Truth authorizes and balances. We might buy enough time to gain a handle on world conditions so perilous and precarious that the very survival of the human race is in question.

Many people today around the world feel completely surrounded, outgunned, and outmaneuvered by North Atlantic secular military-industrial culture; the main sacred ideal by which they live is to die in killing us. The secularized age that spreads electronically hither, thither, and yon has left most of us incapable of grasping the tremendous residual power of religious belief, the compelling anthem of faith, and the power of ritual experienced as sacred. We dangerously fail to grasp the cultural mindset of our enemies, whether Islamic extremists or our own religious extremists. Theater, whether musical or not, can help us grasp the white-hot fusions into groups that mightily empower their members. Because performers, composers, directors, and audience are the creators of performance art, they interweave in the most intimate way with each other, disclosing our shared life, our mimetic engulfment in each other—what is so taken for granted that it cannot typically be questioned by us because it is just "the way things are."

Each interweaving partner is a creating center that discerns aspects, sides, crevices that the others can't discern, given the limits of each point of view. When these creators pool together these discerned features in a performance or rehearsal, something of the shape, limits, rhythms, direction, and pulse of their shared life in the world emerges.[2] This emergence is signaled by a peculiar silence of rapt attention in which we barely breathe, even in a secular age. The moments of disclosure emerge from a

2. The discovery of so-called mirror neurons in the brain is of the greatest significance. It happened somewhat accidentally in the 1990s. Very fine electrodes had been inserted in a baboon's brain to monitor circuits in its behavior—for example, when it ate. One hot day, while a lab assistant was eating an ice cream cone within the baboon's direct experience, sounds from the monitor were emitted identical to those that occurred when the baboon itself was eating. The encrusted paradigm of psychophysical dualism inherited from Descartes—which carried the corollary assumption that mental events are private and personal—was burst open. The discovery opened the door to a flood of accumulating empirical findings. Briefly, we participate as bodies in each other's "interior mental life"; we are social creatures to a degree unimagined by most thinkers previously. Even others' intentions to do something are immediately shared by us to a significant degree, as these will be experienced as our *own* potentialities. Much more beckons to be learned about all this; For example, why are some intentions never acted out? (I imagine that modes of the frontal cortex's inhibitory powers must be discovered.) But one clear consequence is that the role of direct, immediate, face-to-face contact with others contributes most powerfully to our socialization and general development as persons. This is not centrally a matter of sharing abstract data, knowledge *about* things, or even pictures. It is direct, immediate, and engulfing bodily *acquaintance*. See also Appendix B on the brain.

level beneath that of prosaic verbal speech. I think we should regard them as numinous and sacred in some real sense (see Wilshire, *Role Playing and Identity: The Limits of Theatre as Metaphor*, especially Chapter 6). I think the term *sacred* should be used in this connection.

We have taken at least a step toward becoming our own chorus. If we understand that this is *our* white-hot fusion and authorization, then the other foreign group must have its own white-hot fusion, one that is often barely grasped by them, and probably never grasped by us. By understanding this, we are loyal to the truth of our actual experiencing and true to the earth, as Nietzsche put it, and similarly Emerson: "Speak the truth, . . . and the very roots of the grass underground there do seem to stir and move to bear you witness" (*Nature and Selected Essays*, 110). If this rings true to us—particularly in our chests, hearts, lungs, bowels—we have taken a step in a learning process that might yet buy enough time to hold off planetary catastrophe, perdition. We might actually become the last best hope of earth. Farfetched? Perhaps. But as William James put it, there may be no hope, but if we don't hope there is certainly none.

It is strange to think that we must heartily and courageously explore our own bodies. "If they get us around well enough we must already know them!" No, not necessarily. We are aware at various times and in various ways. But we are aware *organisms*. These organisms generate awareness under various conditions. Yet the awareness generated need not be aware of these generating conditions in the organism and environment. In fact, our early conditioning at the hands of caregivers may have disinclined us to explore our own bodies from within our bodies, because this is typically of such little interest to others. Or they may have actively discouraged our own potential interest because of their prudish ideas about the body. "No, we are really nonbodily souls or minds that just happen to have a body in this life."

Very early we fell into line mimetically and automatically with those looming others around us, what they could know of us, what they called us, what they demanded of us, how they conditioned us in our nervous systems. We congealed into habits and probably deadening trances, very like being hypnotized. Other possible ways of being became masked out, and then this masking was itself masked out. The ultimate occlusion is that we don't know that there is much we don't know; we can't even suspect its possibility. We exist in very bad trance, very serious boredom, or exercising futile and frantic attempts to escape these.

Many are, I believe, buried alive—in a real sense—with only the faintest vibrations from the world out there, or even from their own organism in here, reaching them. On the whole, secularized people today, though they may insist that their lives are solid and sure, have never shouted a secret to the stone—or done its equivalent, whatever that might be. They haven't realized viscerally that we share our matter with the stone, and that there are unimagined reaches of the unknown, unimagined reaches of what we don't know that we don't know. They lack any shred of the sacred, that numinous sense of what's greatly good, indeed what's unconditionally valuable and powerful for all us beings, human and nonhuman.

To open up new horizons and locate friendly winds for our explorations and navigations, we must in fact get to know our own bodies: how they resonate in one way or another with things, or fail to do so. Also, how they resonate within themselves, or fail to do so. We are not machines but rather, when healthy, are growing organisms in which like engenders like unwittingly and fluidly. When released from fixations, we are musical body-minds, body-selves—fugal, flowing, interweaving, shifting, opening and closing structures and patterns. We can exist well only when rhythmically sipping or gulping life's fluid power. The power is there, only typically hidden by the endless deadening hype and frenzy of the technologized and commercialized culture, a heedless and superficial materialism. When we open ecstatically to the cosmos—to the more than we can imagine—we feel whole and become so.

Performance arts can, in pregnant moments, put us in touch with our body-minds and body-selves; even poets composing alone may be reciting and chanting as they write. The trick is to stay in touch with our bodily selves in their most concrete detail after the performance is finished and we file out again into the street and back to the dailyness of life. A pioneer in this field of body exploration was F. M. Alexander, a performer who suffered fixations or hang-ups in his body that impeded his performance and that he patiently deciphered. Another pioneer was Ida Rolf, who discovered ways of kneading and freeing up the sheaths of the muscles, the fascia, that constrict our muscles and confine our muscle-memory, so that new possibilities for being and acting are blocked. Another is Moshe Feldenkrais, a polymath who discovered greatly original, ecstatic, and imaginative departures and horizons for explorations of the body—the body as we immediately live it in its interior darkness, not just the body as an object for science (as important as that is). All these pioneers discovered insidious limits on our freedom in the way we lived in our bodies, on our freedom to change, and helped to soften the barriers and limits, and perhaps to move through them.

Feldenkrais, influenced by philosopher-psychologist Maurice Merleau-Ponty and possibly also by William James, was a particularly intrepid, patient, discerning explorer who confronted his body-self's disabilities unflinchingly. Most basically he had absorbed the insights of Romantics of the early nineteenth century. The body is not a mechanism; it is an organism. If part of a mechanism fails, this does not necessarily involve all the other parts of the machine; often the failed part can be replaced and the machine will work well again. But in an organism, each part so deeply and instantaneously resonates with all the others that if a member fails, that failure will ramify through the whole organism, perhaps also bringing on failures in apparently remote organs. The much-at-once often comes in engulfing, overwhelming, dissonant chords.

Most specifically, each member or part of an organism resonates not only with the immediate whole, the particular body in question, but with the universe, even if unwittingly. Each whole is a whole of parts, and each whole is in turn part of a larger whole, and so on toward the limit. Similitudes and kinships emerge in the most unexpected places, finding echoes and resonances where the merely verbal intellect cannot follow. *Simul in multis*. The whole universe sings, as Pythagoras of Samos heard and exclaimed long ago. For Charles Peirce the basic assumption must be continuity. Only when there is good reason to believe in separation should we believe it.

At a fairly advanced period of his life, Feldenkrais developed such spasms in his lower trunk and legs that he walked with a limp. For hours he explored, groping with his body-mind through the dark reaches and vastnesses of his body—a body that was struggling to understand itself from within itself. He felt his way through regions of his own body, experiencing what few people have imagined. He somehow intuited a connection between the movements of his eyes—and the muscles activating them—and the muscles in spasm in his lower trunk and legs. He found that if he relaxedly opened and dilated his eyeballs and their muscles, the anal and urethral sphincters also relaxed slightly. He began opening his mouth and "sloppily" kissing his forearm, exploring the mouth as sphincter. Again, the excretory sphincters also opened and relaxed slightly, which resonated with his ambulatory muscles, which freed him from the limp. The eyes as sphincters! That puts vision in its place without losing it in the process.

Ecstatically exploring his body, not as an object but as immediately lived from within, Feldenkrais released himself from an otherwise intractable fixation.

One of Feldenkrais's first students, Ruthy Alon, spoke of the chest as the "toughest nut to crack": toughest in terms of locating its constrictions, its cemented habits that shut down growth and the fluid unfolding of the person's deepest capacities, that ruin the person's musicality. The whole trunk (including the abdomen) is most interior, most difficult to focus and get a purchase on, most completely implicit and taken for granted. How do we recognize and treat our fixations lodged there? How do we achieve a new reach of actual freedom?

This is tied in with another profound problem, one that William James recognized in the later nineteenth century. How do we do something for the first time? How are we greatly creative? To act voluntarily, we need the sensations and muscle-and-nerve memories left by previous bodily activities. In acting we anticipate their reoccurrence; however, the efferent, descending—or "commanding"—neural system generates no afferent or ascending sensations that might be retained (or only exceedingly subtle ones). Since we must use such retained sensations to act in a certain way, how can we do something for the first time? How can we be free?

Well, we can understand *that*. Feldenkrais did understand that. If he detected a hang-up deep in his trunk, he would manipulate that area with his hands, knead it at certain depth and in a certain direction that felt right, liberating. He would tap a hidden and blocked tendency or nisus toward health. If this kneading of the trunk succeeded, it left deposits of sensations retained in his primary memory. These, when anticipated, would provide material necessary for voluntary actions—ones based in his own initiative—without the aid of his hands kneading his trunk. *Voila!* Freedom, real agency as whole persons.

In the face of previously unheard of dangers, we can detect new networks of communication—perhaps of communion—forming in various regions of the planet. New initiatives are emerging within and between some groups that had previously been cemented in their divergent and antagonistic ways (for example, international meetings on Interdependency Day). These initiatives are often nascent. We will have to listen as patiently and acutely as did Native Americans with their ears to the ground. We will have to develop our awareness of our own proprioceptive or kinesthetic reality as members of groups, and do so as patiently as Moshe Feldenkrais intuited connections between the sphincter-like movements of his eyes and various movements in his trunk and lower body. Otherwise, all our talk of a new reach of freedom across the board is just blather, self-congratulation and self-deception.

Centers of creativity will have to counterbalance in some way neoconservative ideologues in our United States, who feel fine about perpetuating colonialism in new guises, who often confuse it with "God's plan"; to counterbalance, also, Muslim and other extremists whose main meaning in life is to kill others along with themselves. Can we fall in love again with life? Might this love be contagious, be caught even by our enemies? With its infinite variety, never fully predictable, can life itself be received and accepted as a gift infinitely precious, infinitely beyond price and calculation, and ecstatically shared? Can we take initiatives to drain the hellholes of the world? The refugee camps, the squalor, disease, ignorance, and hopelessness, much of it beyond eyeshot perhaps, but to which we might *hearken* and take action?

Could it be that the survival of the planet's life may depend upon our being morally good—and being perceived to be so? An account of a twenty-seven-year-old Palestinian attorney, a woman who served as a suicide bomber, exemplifies the relevance yet the insufficiency of scientific explanations. Many of the deficiencies of the Palestinians' situations may be measurable ones of food, shelter, clothing, mobility, health and educational services, and so on. Ingredient in this woman's motivations is a sense of a deficiency of justice. To speak of a deficiency of justice, however, is only a manner of speaking, is it not? No definite numbers can be placed on this deficiency, nor on how its felt sense impacts her whole spiritual-mental-physical life at a particular moment. Who could possibly predict when a sense of injustice will, in any individual case, break the threshold and be acted out? There is no way to judge how inflamed and agonized is a person's primal sense of right and wrong, those basal felt meanings—the bass notes—in one's troubled world-as-experienced. To feel unjustly treated, decade after decade, is to feel that something sacred has been desecrated.

Can we become more inventive in what we pick out to perceive? I ask myself, can I perceive that fundamentalists of all sorts—Christian, Jewish, Muslim, neoconservative ideologues and free-marketers—are the most dangerous groups on the planet, but also that they too are terrified of the unknown and of their vulnerability? If I am poised, balanced, a bit loose in the joints, I will be less apt to clutch up in panic when encountering strange human beings—that is, ones who act strangely because they experience the world quite differently from the way I or my group does. That is, they live within a much-at-once in which their culture has selected certain things for their attention, and has selected others to be ignored. They live a world-as-experienced quite different from my own.

If I retain my poise in the face of the strange, I will have found my music that is right for me to flourish in the world. If I succeed in doing this, I will tolerate—maybe even learn to enjoy—what is not itself aggressively intolerant. The greater the *multis,* the greater the *simul*, the greater the tension that runs through the *multis*, its vitality, élan. Attuned with the much-at-once, I will be more effective in fiercely defending myself when mortally threatened, because I am more poised and deeply assured. There are of course war dances, chants, songs, but if we are poised and alert we may resonate to the particular dangers of encouraging aggression, war, and genocide in the world as it now precariously stands.

Clearly, in this writing I have selected particular pieces and types of music to emphasize. My penchant is for "classical" music; it has always meant the most to me, meant more than I am able to say, even when I work on saying it. But clearly, the kinds of music that activate and energize others' bodies are greatly various. My music in the broadest and most liberated sense should allow me to flow with all this, even when that requires some initial effort. My music should encourage mutual respect. My music should prompt and release me to dilate my body's organs and my attention, and perhaps pick out and value what is of great value to amazingly various others. *Simul in multis*: myself threading through and allowing, accepting, the many greatly different things all around. This would be the most beneficial weaving imaginable—perhaps a weaving beyond our present capacities to imagine.

A people's music is essential to them. Nietzsche wrote that without music, life would be an error. Just whistling or humming as I work, I am accompanied by a reliable "other," myself as flowing and confident, myself keeping myself in good company. A mother sings her little daughter to sleep each night with a lullaby: her breathing slows as she settles trustingly into the arms of slumber. Her heart, her eyes, her whole body-self is assured that she can lose consciousness without incurring danger. An Islamic school child in mountainous upper Pakistan spins out the ancient complicated scales of his region on a traditional stringed instrument and feels perfectly at home, welcome, in the funded life of his people. An Aboriginal in the Australian interior evokes the spirits and myriad kin with the earthen sounds and pulses of the didgeridoo—a marvelous instrument, not just "a crude wooden trumpet," as one anthropologist described it. Africans communicate across great distances with their drums, and commune with the many pulses of life. All the various musics of the incredibly various human race.

How is it with our souls? Ah, *soul.* We needn't always avoid the word! It needn't connote that putatively nonphysical part of us that is imagined to survive death. That cannot be proved, and *that* shouldn't bother us. I am completely agnostic on this metaphysical issue. When I speak of "soul" I refer to something palpably, sensuously evident—though not easily described or encompassed. As stated, I mean all that the *body* does, and I mean also what we cannot now imagine the whole body might do. I don't ignore the eyes. Even the old saw, eyes as windows of the soul, can be redeemed. Eyes can reveal what one is inclined to do, one's deep potentialities.

I believe that when the strands of music, science, ecstasy, the body are heard, seen, felt dilatedly and penetratingly within the much-at-once in which we live, we will gain insight into what the soul demonstrably *is*. On my view, the soul is not another strand to be woven. *It is our whole being resonating with what is bounteously and magnanimously sacred.* Here I employ the distinction that William James used to distinguish "knowledge by description" from what he called "knowledge by acquaintance." By the latter he meant not just prosaically verbal knowledge *about* something, data, but knowledge as the immediate presencing of something, a *being grasped* by that thing or phenomenon—feeling-fully, viscerally, compellingly, sustainingly. No flash in the pan, it is knowledge as intensity, weight, immediacy, momentousness, the sacred. It is what Beasley experienced anatomizing the viscera of the seal.

LINGERING AFTERWORD

This book is meant to be a progression in intensity. It is not just another linear book, such as a mystery or detective story: First we learn this detail, then that, then another, then finally discover who, say, killed the heiress. Nor is it linear in the way that garden-variety empirical research is so: We learn this fact, then another, then another, and finally discover what causes, say, the carrots to mildew while still growing. As a progression in intensity, the book is more cyclical than linear. To break the benumbed trances of everyday living—particularly the technological trance—I have drawn out some matters in Part I at length, even developing a bit the idea of the eyes as sphincters. When matters are thus drawn out, slowed down—as well as sometimes abruptly developed—the humdrum, benumbed rhythms of everyday life are violated and simultaneously revealed. We may become disenthralled.

In Part II, I sometimes speed up the rhythms and hit them harder and more abruptly still. The point of this is to violate the abysmally routinized and humdrum in startling ways, and thereby to reveal it, to free us from its clutches. How free are we, we who trumpet "Freedom! Freedom!" to the world? The whole of Part II deals with our supposedly distinctive powers of self-reflection as human selves. What is the range and depth of these, really? Are we too limited and finite to realize just how finite we are? I will deal with what many people call the human soul, but will do so without losing sight of the fact that we are organisms evolved within Nature—that we are ineluctably physical, messy, essentially traumatizable creatures capable of endemic self-deception.

Along the way, Part II develops further the power of music and the world of sound to orient, ground, balance, empower us—that is, to reroot and re-enliven our experiencing of the world so that we might be better poised, alert, eager to live, not so incredibly fearful of losing our balance, for fear and weaponry are a substitute ecstasy, a desperate "fix" and filler. Sound and music can reach us from all around ourselves; they, and the metaphors they generate, can work to free us from the compulsive straight-ahead stance and thrust of vision and its metaphors. We fall into humdrum trances easily and experience life as somnambulism, like a troubled and driven sleepwalker. It is extraordinarily difficult to awaken from such trances because to live in a trance is of course not to realize that we are in one. But as long as we are playing and hearing, open to music's power to intrude into and shatter our trance state, we remain confident and able to grow. We are not rushing madly, numbed, obsessed; nor are we bullying or humiliating others, or threatening them with genocide.

Reader, I dared anticipate your attention through this Lingering Afterword. Please accompany me now to Part II.

PART TWO

MUSIC, ART, SCIENCE, GENIUS

Helplessness in their chests is what steers their wandering minds.

—Heraclitus

The human species is the . . . most immature, newest species. . . . We have only just arrived. If we can continue our questioning, our developing . . . if we can live in awe and in the depths of wonder, we will continue moving into the only process that now matters—our authentic maturation as a species.

—Brian Swimme

SEGMENT FIVE

FUGAL STRANDS TO BE WOVEN

As I wrote in the Lingering Afterword to Part I, elongating and slowing down rhythms can throw routine, everyday patterns into relief, can reveal them. What is ordinarily engulfed, dulled, hidden can be prized out and examined. Specifically, following Feldenkrais, vision has been moved out of the hierarchical and dualistic picture—eyes as "windows of the soul"—to also being considered among the body's sphincters. This radically recontextualizes and reveals.

In Nietzsche's last bursts of lucidity, he conveyed insights of incomparable insight and daring. It's as if he knew he had only limited time to strike to the heart of the human condition on the eve of the twentieth century, so there was need to strike hard, fast, and deep. He compared history of his day—in his final days—to an ever-accelerating torrent that is unable to reflect on itself, too afraid to reflect on itself. Moreover, he dared to say that only children believe that we are hybrid beings, bodies as well as immaterial souls or spirits. We adults know that we *are* our bodies (see Wilshire, *Wild Hunger: The Primal Roots of Modern Addiction*, 59). What a daunting prospect to try to work all this out! But if we catch the note of Nietzsche's urgency, we might at least try. Feldenkrais, with his insight that the eyes are sphincters along with the urethral and anal ones, dares to tackle the childish mind/body dualism; he emboldens us to try to be adults and fully inhabit our bodily selves before it is too late.

"Eyes pertain to light and mind, and these are the antipode of urine and feces!" That's the dualistic notion so deeply accepted as to be utterly taken for granted—the subconsciously accepted assumption and norm upon which people attempt to build their lives. Along with Nietzsche, Feldenkrais shakes this foundation of people's experienced world and offers some possibility that we will wake up from somnambulism. Or is it that, in a real sense, we are buried alive, as I suggested earlier? It is next to impossible to overestimate the significance of the connections that Nietzsche and Feldenkrais discern in the body—the body-self or body-mind—or, as we shall see, in the mind of music. One can be crippled for a lifetime by the condemning look of the other, branded into one's sentient body early in life. Indigenous peoples—for example, in India—speak of this as "the evil eye." Thus they thematize it for us and rescue it from the oblivion of fastidious Western mind/body dualism, with its repression and forgetfulness of the body. Feldenkrais saw that all the sphincters are connected organismically, so that if one is changed, all the others are also. Indeed, the whole body is interconnected organismically in its whole neuromuscular-skeletal anatomy. If a person is frozen in terror early in life by the other's evil-making eye, the victim will keep staring into the eyes of the other, trying helplessly to ward them off. This is counterproductive, however, as it locks up one's whole bodily adaptive system—which is really one's *minding* system.

So Feldenkrais proposes a simple countermeasure. Given that one's eyes have been frozen by the trauma, immobilized in consequence of their own venturing in the world, they have in effect become "locked" into the head, remaining stationary, being moved only through the head's movement. Feldenkrais devises floor exercises that systematically and ritualistically turn the eyes in a direction oblique to the way the head faces, in tension with the torso, so they become unlocked; once thus freed, the eyes are empowered to lead the head and the torso's movements. Instead of the eyes being "carried along" with the body and the head's movements, their directedness begins to determine the movement of the body. In this way the eyes can be trained to lead the body in new freeing movements, instead of being passive receptacles, and the visual field correspondingly becomes much expanded.

We have a wide range of voluntary control over the eyes that we do not with other sphincters. Instead of the eyes being shackled, they can free themselves and the rest of the body-self. Since all the sphincters are interconnected organismically, a violation of the eyes may well involve also a violation of the anal sphincter. The whole body-self may be frozen in fear of, say, anal penetration. The victim might suffer homosexual nightmares, but with no repressed desire for homosexual lovemaking (if so, a qualification of Freud's universal wish-fulfillment theory would be called for: The root of behavior and being would in certain cases be terror, not sexual desire).

One way to break up the trance, to bring the benumbed rhythms of everyday life to focal awareness is to create contrast: to elongate and slow down the rhythms, as I tried to do in the preceding segment. Another way, which I take now, is to break in on them with swift, bold strokes—to compress them—and to do so close to home. Close to home in our own bodies, of course, but also close to home in our United States, citing cases of well-known Americans, all of them irruptive geniuses. I allude to geniuses not to be absorbed in their "personalities" but to benefit from their irruptive creativity as we struggle for real freedom. Standing on tiptoe as dancers might, they glimpse new horizons and fresh angles on things. Through their imagining as bodily beings, they assume new standpoints and throw matters into revealing new contexts. Creativity: the spontaneous constructing of comprehension, the play that is serious. The great challenge remains: to become our own chorus, our own detachment within our involvements, our own reality-check, to shake ourselves loose from humdrum deadening trance into the ecstatic trance of true creativity.

Kant's definition of genius is as good as any: a person who cannot live within the received assumptions, norms, and rules and creates new ones that are productive of insight. For my purposes I pick out for special attention Thomas Jefferson, Ralph Waldo Emerson, and Charles Sanders Peirce. The first and the last of these were deranged by their disruptive defiance of embedded public norms, at least to the point of experiencing incapacitating migraine headaches for weeks on end, not to mention that they often baffled even their own supporters. Then there is Emerson, poet and philosopher, who so expanded the scope and pull of learning, yet he observed that it was the learned classes who offered the most stubborn resistance to exploration and growth. (Alfred North Whitehead similarly remarked that the overconfidence of learned people is the comic tragedy of civilization.)

One could argue, of course, that all the revolutionists, the patriots of 1776, were disruptive geniuses, for they defied the generally accepted assumption of their times that humans cannot govern themselves. It was commonly thought that humans need a royal ruler garbed in God's authority to provide a head for the corporate bodies of human groups; whereas for the revolutionary patriots the United States would become the great experiment, and they staked their lives on its success. I opt, however, to limit the discussion to my three exemplars of genius. When just a very few notable and homegrown individuals forcibly depart from deeply accepted norms, they can shake us into a new level of wakefulness, I believe. They can join the ranks of more distant exemplar individuals, such as the Buddha, who bore the name that means "the one who awakened."

This second part of the book takes a fresh approach to exposing how taken-for-granted, deeply encrusted, vision-dominated assumptions, concepts, distinctions, rhythms, and norms limit, constrict, and benumb thought and behavior. It will now proceed with an unaccustomed brevity and abruptness, as I hope that a few well-aimed blows from unexpected angles will loosen the rust on these ways of thinking and being. Constant and contrastless, they are no longer noticed. But if we learn to hear their humdrum rhythms *as* humdrum, we might then break their grip. We would no longer sleepwalk.

Each human group sorts out the multifarious events of experience in its distinctive way. As a group habitually sorts out the world—categorizes, classifies, names—so to a huge extent it *is*. What sorts of things are to be noticed? What sorts downplayed or ignored—or tabooed? How much is to be made of any given kind of event? How is a world built up in experience? This customary selectivity and construction within the streaming barrage of experience is so habitual and so completely taken for granted that few in the group are aware of what is going on. For most, this mindless everyday consensus concerning what is to be noticed, what ignored, comprises what the world *is*. We can call these persons naive realists. For them, confronting an assertive foreign culture is somewhat baffling—even, in certain unsettled circumstances, terrifying. The foreigners clearly experience things quite differently from the way "we" do, yet they seem to get on well enough!

The seeds of a corrosive self-doubt may be implanted in members of the home group. The very solidity of things as they are directly experienced by these members may give way beneath their feet (see Wilshire, *Get 'Em All! Kill 'Em!: Genocide, Terrorism, Righteous Communities*). I believe that groups that commit genocide are as terrified in their way as groups subjected to genocide are in theirs. The everyday consensus within the home group concerning reality is not just "in the mind"; it permeates whole body-selves caught up in mimetic contagion with others in their group. We should call it intercorporeality: shared perceptual stances; shared expectations built into nervous systems; shared attentions and inattentions; shared rhythms, aversions, disgusts, and bubbling elations. So constantly does this consensus, this humdrum agreement, repeat and reinforce itself that we should talk not merely of the humdrum but of the *group trance*.

The latter half of the eighteenth century inaugurated what is well named the Age of Revolution. A significant portion of tradition was turned on its head and shaken to pieces. That is, traditional group trance was broken to a considerable extent along many parameters. Peculiar universal geniuses stepped in to create new ways of experiencing, new ways of ordering and assembling the world-experienced. Yet we must realize, I believe, that to break down the old trances and try to start afresh, they were caught up in *countertrances*. Old magical incantations and charms were attacked with new ones, however unable the geniuses may have been to acknowledge what they were doing. Old patterns of behavior enshrining sacred, mythic power were to be replaced by new patterns, new enshrinements, new rhythms, melodies, harmonies, structures of experiencing. That was the intention.

In order to try to grasp the situation in which the United States first began to form, we must look back through the intervening almost two hundred fifty years. During this time the United States became the planet's most powerful nation, as power is typically measured by the yardsticks of our own devising. It is immensely difficult to believe how fragile, chancy, and improbable was the assemblage of bustling revolutionaries in 1776. Among the virtues they exhibited were improvisatory power, imagination, creativity, and courage that challenge description. They were traitors in the eyes of England, then the most powerful nation on earth. But they had staked their lives and their *sacred* honor. They believed in the power of reasoning individuals to order their own lives for the best. Many of the important founders were not Christians, but they believed that "Nature's God" had created each of us with certain inalienable and sacred rights to think for ourselves and to take responsibility for our personal and corporate conduct.

To think that the world can be started over again from scratch is absurd, yet the Age of Revolution did bite deep into traditional ways of experiencing and acting. A king, queen, or pope could no longer function unquestionably as God's representative on earth, occupying the center around which all human affairs would gravitate in orbit. The people could and must enact and conform to laws that they themselves created. The Enlightenment's "rationality" and brash "this-worldism" opened the way for the progressive secularization of the world, as well as excesses of traditional institutions of authority that in many ways may have led to their own undoing, as Nietzsche sees in the church's insistence on an authority at odds with its own purpose. The United States leads this sea change, given its far-reaching powers, particularly in its later, heavy influence through electronic media in our current world situation. Think only of the power of Hollywood and of advertising to shape viewers' expectations and desires, to shape their world-experienced, no matter where they happen to live.

We are not minds or souls that just happen to be attached to bodies; rather, we are sentient bodies that experience in certain ways. Moreover, we are essentially tool-using and sign-using bodies, and this now includes use of manifold electronic tools. So caught up are we in our newly shaped world-experienced, indeed, that we tend to look right through our revelatory and shaping tools themselves: They are extensions of our various limbs and organs, our hands, and are as unnoticed as these are when all is working hummingly. Our tools and signs use us as much as we use them—that is, they generate consequences, most of which we cannot begin to encompass or envisage in our consciousness.

The meaning of anything includes *all* the consequences of that thing. But so taken with "consciousness" are we that we tend to be heavily preoccupied with the consequences of acts and events that we are able to grasp in our consciousness. But that is only a middling portion of the full consequences. The meaning of what we are doing today is largely hidden from us, caught up as we are in matters that cannot be encompassed in conscious thought or language. We need a more deeply involving, visceral, vibratory awareness—let's call it an inertial music-like awareness—that carries forward to the long-run consequences of things, consequences that exceed what it can grasp consciously, in prosaic words, at any moment. Of course, we are also caught up in those consequences of our electronic tool-use that we *can* grasp: gross immediate power and profit, immediate comfort and convenience. A "state of mind" arises in which we can actually believe that "time is money," whether we acknowledge this explicitly or not. Any time that is not devoted to gaining gross immediate ends tends to be ignored or devalued—considered mere recreation or diversion. Immediate commercial values dominate, even with regard to what gets published and what does not.[1]

Human beings in all cultures have faced the challenge of holding their lives together through time. They devised special days, holy days, in which persons would dilate their awareness and reclaim their roles as tiny but

1. To witness how immediate commercial values dominate in publishing, there is no need to focus on the apparently endless prurient, sensationalistic, and escapist publications. Perhaps more telling is what has happened in the seemingly more intelligent and informative publishing sector through what might be called the "Random Housing" of the world. The values of gripping and easy reading pervade even this sector, with rare exceptions. One might think, given that the large commercial publishing houses make so much money on most of their trade books, they would voluntarily subsidize a few important, difficult books. But this would be naive in the extreme. In our culture of consumption—indeed, rapid consumption and quick turnover—purveyors of print must produce an easily identifiable commodity. Readers must be conditioned to expect an easy and gripping read from nearly every product of that publishing house. Even a good, informative book such as Russell Shorto's *The Island at the Center of the World* (New York: Doubleday, 2004) doesn't require readers to confront and question basic assumptions about what constitutes the vitality of a group, what constitutes a fact, what meaning, truth, beauty are, what the good life is, what time is, and so on. This requires the *work* of thought. Because basic philosophical and ideological biases are never exposed and evaluated, the current ideological battles that threaten the very existence of civilized life on this planet are not confronted and grasped. We might respond with a *ho-hum*, but it's not a *ho-hum* matter.

special beings in the cosmos. They would re-experience their roles as descendants of revered forebears, for example. Spaces and times were cleared for these ancestors to reappear, to have presence here and now again. But even such "special times" can become routinized, so that if they awaken us at all, we still remain within the engrained and benumbing assumptions of the group trance. Thomas Berry has written aptly of the technological trance that prevails today, pervading our military-industrial-commercial-entertainment world. Our secularized life is largely encompassed by the relentless clockwork, the pounding of mechanisms of all sorts: from calendar deadlines for getting children into the "best" preschools (if they would get into the "best" universities), to the noisy ubiquity of machinery itself, to the constant babble of TV with nobody perhaps really watching or listening—the posturing and posing of TV personalities who have no awareness of us, the persons watching. This constant ticking and pounding becomes "normal," tends no longer to be articulately noticed or noted. But it has its effects, particularly when countertrances of holy days are no longer available or really effective. This is not a beat or rhythm of a music that engages and makes alert, but is rather the benumbing effect of a mechanical sort of time marking.

For many today, this sense of the presence of ancestors, say, is completely occluded: Its very possibility is not imagined. Our actual experiencing life tends to shrink and wither. Manifold addictions appear—workaholism, say—attempts to jumpstart us into an eagerness to live. But the body is not rested at those periodic intervals originally determined by the recuperative rhythms of the Nature in which we were formed over many, many millennia, and which most traditional rituals celebrated. The body is violated, and the violations have consequences, whether they are grasped or not. For many, all this seems to be too simple to be true, but what if it *is* true?

In the age of revolutions—simply considering for the moment science and technology—ways of living change rapidly, sweeping our bodily engagement up into this relentless beat, such that it becomes difficult for the musical dimension of our lives to pull us out of this accelerating pace to rediscover other rhythms attuned to dimensions of existence outside this relentless productivity. To believe that we are real, really this or really that, and to become aware of this reality is, I think, the most fundamental of our human needs. Apparently paradoxically, some even sacrifice their very lives to meet it. Think of suicide bombers or, less sensationally, of people who literally work themselves to death in their jobs to win a sense of personal identity and social status they would otherwise feel themselves to be utterly lacking.

Our American founders could not have imagined the effects of our contemporary technologies, industries, and commerce, or the astounding speed with which secularization has taken hold. But I want to focus on those founding persons in our experimental nation who did foretell to some extent the disastrous consequences of mindless secularism; here I consider Jefferson, Emerson, and Peirce as exemplary. Only the first is widely known today, and in only the smallest fragment of his reality. So closeted in contemporaneity are we as a culture (I borrow words from T. S. Eliot) that most academics and scholars today do not really grasp their importance, not even those academics explicitly responsible for keeping us alive to our past traditions and the possibilities they seed.

The need to *be*. Our three thinkers agree that it cannot be met by relying solely on science, technology, and Enlightenment rationalism—the calculating secular mind of *homo economicus*. Required is the retrieval of another dimension of ecstatic living, of perceiving, thinking, interacting, acting. Call it the *sacred* dimension, though as we have seen, it is a vague, slippery, and dangerous yet vital term. The sacred does not belong to a dimension "beyond" this world but rather pertains to the depths of this world as an echo of our species' primordial creation of itself in Nature: our lives as hunter-gatherer-scavengers who were attuned to Nature in a way that eludes us today.

It was in the third year of Jefferson's first term as president of the United States that the philosopher and poet Emerson was born. He was an undistinguished student at Harvard, not yet in command of his gifts. It was not until the publication of the essay "Nature" when he was thirty-three years old that he came into his own. So forcibly and eloquently did he do so that quite a few others in the nineteenth century were able to deeply identify with his writings, with passages such as this:

> The charming landscape which I saw this morning is indubitably made up of some twenty or thirty farms. Miller owns this field, Locke that, and Manning the woodland beyond. But none of them owns the landscape. There is a property in the horizon which no man has but he whose eye can integrate all the parts, that is, the poet. This is the best part of these men's farms, yet to this their warranty-deeds give no title. (*Nature and Selected Essays*, 38)

Ecstatically grasping the horizon—what is actually given us to experience—is crucial for Emerson. The horizon is like the Roman god Janus: two heads pointing in opposite directions: the horizon "on this side" presents itself as enclosing all that might be *directly experienced* by us now, while on "the opposite side," it points beyond all this to *everything else* in the universe, whether ever experienced or not. A moment's thought discloses that, very probably, there are things going on in the universe that we cannot imagine, so cannot imagine to look for.

If we perceive dilatedly, sympathetically, ecstatically—with our hearts as well as our eyes—we realize that sensuous experience leads us beyond even itself. Moreover, this limitless cosmos is where we organisms are really at home and where we belong. It draws us and calls to us, though it is easily drowned out. It is something most "dear and connate" ("Nature," 39); it is something as beautiful as our own nature. Despite forces moving in on us from every side to stamp us into conformity, we are exploratory beings, even as our earliest hunter-gatherer ancestors were. In fact, resonances of their existence still sound within us—sound in a kind of eternal present, an eternal present tense. There is a nisus to *story* this in our various arts. Yes, it may be nearly obliterated in today's benumbing celebrity culture, but for some this nisus is a living root of possibility.

So much for the supposed ultimacy of the contracted present, and for the ultimacy of *homo economicus*, ever striving—even to the death—for easily measured and widely recognized gain. In *The Varieties of Religious Experience*, William James develops this as the peculiar and abiding sense of "the whole residual cosmos that everyone possesses," if they could but acknowledge the gift. Linear time can loosen its grip on us—that obsessive rushing down the addictive tunnel, the dreadful sense of running out of time. We become aware of the cosmos as "circular power returning into itself," ever regenerating of itself; Emerson divinizes it as the "inexplicable continuity of this web of God" in which no manmade deadlines can hold ("The American Scholar" in *Nature and Selected Essays*, 85). The secret is the countertrance of ever-repeated holy days, ones that are prevented somehow from becoming dulled and routine. The secret is to find newly *regenerative* repetitions, those that evoke ecstatically the one throbbing whole: the past, the present, and the domain of undemarcatable possibility—and small as we are, we directly experience that we are a part of it all. Our irruptive geniuses can awaken us to how creatively and arrestingly fugal we can be.

In his essay "Poetry and Imagination" Emerson writes, "We are lovers of rhyme and return. . . . The babe is lulled to sleep by the nurse's song. Sailors can work better for their *yo-heave-o*" ("Poetry and Imagination," 8:24). In the information age it is good to be reminded that Emerson is talking about the vitality of life itself, our reality as ecstatic beings whose lives are woven up fugally and—let us hope—excitedly through time. For information and information theory, repetition is mere clogging redundancy. For poetry, song, myth of all ages, repetition is the charm that counteracts the dispersive and disintegrative power of linear time and lives of mere routine. The only transcendence of linear time possible is *in* time. Some traditional repetitions and incantations are these:

> "Yo-heave-o . . . yo-heave-o . . ." repeated until the rowing is done.
>
> Homer: "rosy-fingered dawn . . . rosy-fingered dawn." Or, "wily Odysseus . . . wily Odysseus . . ."
>
> Albert Camus: "the sky, the earth, the eternal things."
>
> The Finnish epic *Kalevala*: "reckless Lemminkainen . . . reckless Lemminkainen . . ." Or, "O craftsman Ilmarinen . . . O craftsman Ilmarinen . . ." Or, "Steadfast old Vainamoinen . . . Steadfast old Vainamoinen . . ." And on and on, with whole blocks of resonant stanzas repeated again and again, as if in an ongoing chorus of words, an anthem that is a litany in which the whole group as chorus can participate.
>
> Or in the Christian antiphonal: "World without end . . . World without end . . . Amen . . . Amen . . ."

Names do not merely refer to a particular person, but signal the *presence* of the person, evoke it, along with all those beings who are kindred to him or her. Repeated names repeatedly and reliably evoke this accumulating and radiating presence (see John Minahan, *Word Like a Bell: John Keats, Music, and the Romantic Poet*). A bell reverberates and possesses overtones in a way that a string plucked or struck does not; such a power of music intones in our speech and writing. Emerson anchors the universality of song and poetry in the human organism itself. His words cannot be revisited too often:

> Metre begins with pulse-beat, and the length of lines in songs and poems is determined by the inhalation and exhalation of the lungs. If you hum or whistle the rhythm of the common English metres . . . you can easily believe these metres to be organic, derived from the human pulse, and to be therefore not proper to one nation, but to mankind. I think you will . . . be at once set on searching for the words that can rightly fill these vacant beats. ("Poetry and Imagination," 8:24–25)

It is tempting to connect trance with hypnotism, as the two are induced by repetition, but here I decline the opportunity. Suffice it to say that trance comes in many varieties, a multitude that comparison with hypnotism might obscure. Trance can be regenerative when it is evoked by ceremony that dilates awareness or absorption in a task or event that takes us beyond ourselves, or it can be degenerative or indeterminate, as the ones we have explored in mechanized culture; I'm not so sure about hypnotism by contrast, which is our artificially induced attempt to switch the mind into another register.

The verses of Li Po (d. 762) read,

> Flocks of birds have flown high and away,
> A solitary drift of cloud, too, has gone, wandering on.
> And I sit alone with Ching-Ting Peak, towering beyond.
> We never grow tired of each other, the mountain and I.
> ("The Ching-Ting Mountain")

In my own case, I never grow tired of the San Gabriel Mountains of Southern California that accompanied me most of my youth. Part of the reason is that looking at them lovingly means looking carefully, which means noting the endless changes in them. Situations in which they are experienced are never exactly the same—never the same light or atmosphere or wafted fragrance, never quite the same echoes when I shout into their canyons. Moreover, the mountains alter their very surfaces: new vegetation or its demise, new landslides or rockslides after a season of heavy precipitation, and so on.

But beyond all this, mountains are vivid borders and horizons. In showing themselves, they also tacitly reveal that there is that which lies beyond them, what their very presence might hide or obscure to those benumbed in trance: Ultimately it is the *everything else* of the vast and enduring cosmos (see Victor Kestenbaum, *The Grace and the Severity of the Ideal: John Dewey and the Transcendent*). This hints of the loving and perhaps frightening embrace of what we don't know that we don't know. We intuit that this must be infinitely various: It must lie beyond all cataloguing. It must forever lure and excite the human hunter. The mountain and I never grow tired of each other. This is the never failing joy of ever-repeated ecstatic expansion and participation. However dampened and stolid we may become, we are hunters still—the potent call of our species' past remains, as does the underlying thrill of danger.

What kind of thinking is all this? It is *not* the thinking that arose so mightily with the scientific-technological-industrial-commercial revolutions of the seventeenth and eighteenth centuries, envisioning the goals of domination and control of Nature and devising means for achieving them. Man the economic animal, depicted as tyrannical by Robert Marshall: "There is just one hope of repulsing the tyrannical ambition of civilization to conquer every niche on the whole earth. That hope is the organization of spirited people who will fight for the freedom of the wilderness" ("The Problem of the Wilderness," 148). This thinking *is* laying oneself open, heart and mind, to the ancient influences of Nature that formed and still form us, fight and repress them as we may—the much-at-once from every side, angle, level. As we have just seen, Emerson writes of the "*inexplicable* continuity of this web of God" (my emphasis). There is too much going on every moment to presume to place it within the focus of the calculating and theorizing consciousness. The way of life is by abandonment:

> The one thing which we seek with insatiable desire is to forget ourselves, to be surprised out of our propriety . . . to do something without knowing how or why. . . . Nothing great was ever achieved without enthusiasm. The way of life is wonderful; it is by abandonment. . . . Dreams and drunkenness, the use of opium and alcohol are the semblance and counterfeit of this oracular genius, and hence their dangerous attraction for men. For the like reason they ask the aid of wild passions, as in gaming and war, to ape in some manner these flames and generosities of the heart. ("Circles," in *Nature and Selected Essays*, 238)

To do something without knowing how or why is a way of letting go: a form of trust and entrancement. It is a way of being musically. We allow beats of induction to work on us rhythmically, perhaps rhymingly, in a regenerative repetition that takes us beyond ourselves and our usual round into the deeper rhythms of the natural world underlying the idiosyncratic and cultural.

Without Immanuel Kant we can't imagine the deeper thinking of the age. His central insight is that we can never know Nature "in itself," but only as it passes through the conduits and filters of our living, resonating, minding organisms. Emerson picks this up and radicalizes it still further: "Nature always wears the colors of the spirit" (*Nature and Selected Essays*, 39). We must think *transcendentally.* That is an infinitely slippery term, typically construed as denoting a yearning for that which transcends the mundane world of space and time. Whereas *transcendental* since Kant means just the reverse: It means a probing into, a stabbing into, the assumptions always already at work in *all* our perceiving, thinking, experiencing. And wonder of wonders, these must include the anciently embedded instincts of our animal kin for selecting, assembling, and putting together a world in experience. So far, then, is the special, sacred domain from transcending—or leaving—the earth! In "The Transcendentalist," Emerson writes:

> We have yet no man who . . . trusting to his sentiments, found life made of miracles; who, working for universal aims, found himself fed, he knew not how; clothed, sheltered, and weaponed, he knew not how, and yet it was done by his own hands. Only in the instinct of the lower animals we find the suggestion of the methods of it, and something

> higher than our understanding. The squirrel hoards nuts and the bee gathers honey, without knowing what they do, and they are thus provided for without selfishness or disgrace. (*Nature and Selected Essays*, 245)

Emerson catches himself in a bad trance in "History." So constantly do we Western "minds" intone the liturgy of the great centers of civilization—Rome, Paris, Constantinople, and others—that we fall into a self-hypnotizing beat that walls us up in tunnel vision. We forget our animal kin. Throughout his essay, Emerson assumes that we understand what human figures of the past did because we share their motivations: to make merry, to exact revenge, to understand, and so on. Then on the last page of the essay a terrible second thought stops him in his tracks—as if an evil wind strikes him in the face. How much do we actually grasp of history?

> Is there somewhat overweening in this claim? Then I reject all I have written, for what is the use of pretending to know what we know not? . . . I hold our actual knowledge very cheap. Hear the rats in the wall, see the lizard on the fence. . . . As old as the Caucasian man,—perhaps older,—these creatures have kept their counsel beside him, and there is no record of any word or sign that has passed from one to the other. . . . What a shallow village tale our so-called History is. How many times we must say Rome and Paris, and Constantinople? What does Rome know of rat and lizard? What are Olympiads and Consulates to these neighboring systems of being? ("History," in *Nature and Selected Essays*, 172)

Thus Emerson interrupts himself and confronts a hitherto unsuspected vista. He realizes that our inherited modes of making sense are undermined, are not fundamental. That we are not enclosed and at home in the "family of man," but that we are neighbors to, in fact kin to, the rats in the wall, the lizard on the fence, primitive forms of scurrying, anxious, needy life.

Emerson is sometimes called a pantheist. This misleads, however well intentioned it may be. For a *theist* is one who believes above all in a deity that transcends the mundane world of space and time (even if the deity intervenes in the world in various ways). To say *pan-theist*, then, to say that God is everything, or is identical with Nature, is to utter a self-contradiction.

Calling Emerson a pantheist, however, does have the virtue of disallowing a gulf between the sacred and the secular, thus precluding the possibility that the sacred could fall away and leave the secular standing naked and alone. It is a secular that cannot stand alone since its sources lie in a deeper history entwined with that of the planet; we sense the insubstantiality of being mired in our secular crises without connecting to this deeper, long-term past. Sadly, the subtleties surrounding the notion of pantheism in Emerson are lost on the vast majority of people, who expect simple, hard-and-fast distinctions. We may live in the age of science and technology, but it is also the age of simplisms, numberless oversimplifications, and sclerotic routinized ways.

To call Thomas Jefferson a multifaceted genius would be true, but fails to capture the breadth and depth of the man. Descending in large part from the Enlightenment, he denied claims of Christianity that he regarded as supernaturalistic, unprovable, simpleminded. He was also an ecstatic visionary, and yet his persona as a political leader could not publicly display his greater depths. The resulting instability in his person was essential to his astonishing creativity.[2]

2. In addition to focusing on Jefferson as an example of the instabilities of genius, I might have chosen Alexander Hamilton. The architectural reach and span of his attention, his imagination, was astonishing. Even in his twenties, long before the Constitutional Convention, he had sketched the general structure of the government that would take shape. Genius seems to depend both on this imaginative reach and on the spontaneous inspiration of the moment that occasions the emergence of the sweeping vision. But the two do not always synchronize. Thus at certain moments Hamilton was impulsively and self-damagingly spontaneous. To cite one instance, he wrote a booklet attacking the head of his party and the sitting president of the United States, John Adams, thus nearly insuring that Jefferson, Hamilton's avowed ideological opponent, would be elected in 1800. Were Jefferson elected, Noah Webster wrote to Hamilton, "the fault will lie at your door and . . . your conduct on this occasion will be discerned little short of insanity" (David McCullough, *John Adams*, 550). Why did he do it? "Probably not even Hamilton knew the answer." Historian Ron Chernow, in *Alexander Hamilton*, writes of an "element of ecstatic defiance" in his make-up (115), his ever "shading into excess" (190). Close observers detected "something contradictory in the way the mobile features shifted quickly from gravity to mirth. . . . This mixture of the grave and the playful was the very essence of his nature" (188). Challenged by Aaron Burr to a duel over personal attacks, Hamilton's ability to coordinate the long view and the nearly immediate future seems to have broken down completely. Disagreeing in principle over dueling as an institution, Hamilton may have decided to fire first and to waste his shot. But what could he—a father and husband—have been thinking? That Burr, a seasoned soldier and killer, deeply aggrieved, would do the "chivalrous thing" and not aim to kill him? But why should we assume that he was thinking coherently at all? Isn't it more plausible to assume that he was in the grip of a trance?

Author of the Declaration of Independence, he has aptly been called the poet of the American Revolution. He believed that we were "endowed by our Creator with certain inalienable rights." But this was no mere dry deduction of the creature's rights from the nature of the Creator's acts. Nor were his words "Nature and Nature's God" merely formulaic, a rhetorical gesture; they seem to have had for him the punch of numinousness and sparkling entrancement. He had a vision of self-regulating human beings who could only come into their own through collective, collaborative effort with others in community. This larger body of the community would constitute the proper self-regulating being of the human. A *res publica*—the public's thing—a republic in which each member is educated to realize and believe that what is best for each is what is best for all. A republic is composed of members who respect the laws that they themselves have thoughtfully enacted. Jefferson's Declaration of Independence must be regarded as a kind of musical composition—a striking hymn of praise to human possibilities.

After the revolution he served as special emissary to France. Lured to southern France on holiday, he encountered the ancient Roman city of Nîmes. One early evening he found himself at the wonderfully preserved Roman structure, Maison Carrée, built on the Greek model. I think one should say that this presence induced in him an ecstatic and beneficent trance. What if the Roman republic could live again? What if the advent of the Caesar strong man could be avoided and a true republic be formed and stay alive? Perhaps we should say that Jefferson was as much in tune with the much-at-once as it is humanly possible to be. It was as if he were immersed in water at body-temperature and responsive to every ripple, wave, and current from every side every second—all the while buoyed ecstatically. It may be no accident that Nîmes is the site of ancient waterworks, aqueducts, canals, fountains, pools, and that flowing water has supplied the best metaphor for evoking the flow of our awareness.

William James speaks of the stream of consciousness and James Joyce employs the method of the same name to disclose in words what people live through each moment of every day. "Streaming" suggests not only the flowing of awareness, but glimmering reflections thrown off the stream's surface. These reflections are often fantastical, for evoked are mythic associations from primal sources of humankind within our lineage: reveries and daydreams of dominance and submission, say, or radiant fleeting images of incredible power and potency. But deeper than these visual metaphors are auditory ones. A Chinese Taoist refers to the sound of streaming waters as the sound of prayer. Take the babbling of a brook, and how this suggests the babbling of an infant in the looming protective presence of parents. Evoked, perhaps, are the child's petitions for aid and succor, her rejoicing when soothed, or her gaiety when discovering certain things. All this is retained, I think, in our dreaming and daydreaming life—the benevolent trance life—no matter our age. In hearing music do we partake of this middle ground between sleep and wake? In hearing music do we dream together—and do so beyond the power of linear time to enclose us in mere passing moments? Beyond, as well, the power of understanding—as most people grasp that term? (I contrast "understanding" and "reason" below.) Streaming suggests obscure flows and depths, the numinous reality of *what we don't know that we don't know.* These are the materials of truly ecstatic trance. As Dostoevsky put it, "Nothing is more fantastic than reality itself," particularly the reality of our own immediately experiencing selves embraced, nudged, fed by our own immediately experienced intercirculating world.

As already noted, facile contrasts and oppositions between everyday words very often seduce us to infer that what these words refer to or evoke are simply opposed, as, for example, light to dark, black to white, silence to noise. Thus awake/asleep—how misleading it is! Thus we facilely oppose our productive waking awareness to the supposed idleness of daydreaming, cutting ourselves off from the regenerative power of reverie and imaginative trance. Jefferson seems often to have been powerfully transported in the grip of entrancing visions or variously felt presences. So powerfully, it seems, that he was carried beyond the confines of the everyday consensual reality, the conventional world as experienced by his contemporaries at the time. Did this produce latent anxiety? In any case, Jefferson did in fact pay a heavy price for his transports. He was hungover, racked with exhaustion and incapacitating headaches for weeks after writing the Declaration of Independence. He had been *possessed* by the muses, as the ancient Greeks would describe it (see again E. R. Dodds, *The Greeks and the Irrational*).

There was an omnivorous and cosmic quality to Jefferson's trances and visions. Apparently he was *driven* to place his unique stamp upon the world as he experienced it. So forcibly and eloquently did he stamp it that others were drawn in to experience things that way, at least to the degree they were willing and capable. A notoriously misleading verbal opposition—though we use it in everyday humdrum life—is self/other. In general, people who dominate others through their powerful rhythms, beats, flows, tend to draw others in their wake. Being entranced tends to entrance in turn.

An example of this is Jefferson's purchase of the vast, sparsely mapped Louisiana Territories. He seized the moment when a greatly ambitious Napoleon badly needed money. Jefferson found fifteen million dollars. There was no sanction for this purchase in the United States Constitution, nor was there any general movement among government officials to do it. Jefferson simply did it, and his critics, not completely silent, were left stunned at the barn door: The horse was gone. It was a fait accompli—a prodigy of imagination and daring. (Jefferson sent Lewis and Clark and their comrades to discover just what he had bought. Alarmed, Spanish officials in Santa Fe sent out a large posse to run them down, trailing them by only a week at one point. They did intercept another explorer, Zebulon Pike, returning him to Santa Fe for interrogation. Unable to break him there, they delivered him to Mexico for further torture.)

An immensely insightful observation concerning Jefferson was made by Aaron Burr. This is mediated to us by Gore Vidal in his novel *Burr*, and I take it to be the gist of what Burr said:

> I have not the art to give a proper rendering of his discourse, which came in floods. He seemed to think aloud and, as he did, one was obliged to think with him, in the process becoming so much a part of his mind that each time he hesitated for a phrase, one's own brain stopped all functioning and waited upon his to think for us all, to express for us all. What a devilish gift! (*Burr: A Novel*, 259).

Burr himself felt drawn into Jefferson's rhythmic beat, his entrancing waves of speech. Independent minded and distinctly centered as he was, he remained sufficiently detached to acknowledge and thematize what he experienced. After having experienced its power, he could know the facile opposition self/other was just that: facile and misleading. Others can transport us to realms we wouldn't know, just as the composer does with powerful music.

I've claimed that Jefferson was immersed in the much-at-once and that he was responsive to impulses from every side, but it doesn't follow that he gave balanced responses. He was apt to be carried away in impulse and feeling at particular junctures in his life. It was as if he entranced himself. Thus he was and remained an aesthete, loving beautiful things and beautiful clothes, often spending far beyond his means. A famous portrait shows him as a fur-collared dandy. (Our next genius, Charles Peirce, was also known for his dandyish and spendthrift ways; could it be that the exuberance these two men exhibited in devising novel insights and designs also invaded their more mundane habits?) Yet while he was president, Jefferson affected to look like a common man, sometimes greeting guests at the White House in robe and slippers, so they were not quite sure who he was. Thus his self-dramatizing vision of himself as a yeoman farmer led him to vilify prominent New Englanders as crabbed, closeted in their account books.

This excess led to what most commentators regard as a great blunder in his second term. Responding to British naval intimidation, he and his political followers came up with the Embargo Act of 1807, which shut down ports, particularly in New England. This ultimately precipitated defiance of the law and the near bankruptcy of New England and much of the rest of the nation. Similarly, Jefferson wrote eloquently in the earlier part of his career of the sordid evils of slavery, asserting that it degraded the humanity of both the slave owner and the slave. And yet here again he had to conform to the exigencies of his time and helped fashion the notorious three-fifths clause: In determining representation in Congress, three-fifths of an owner's slaves were to count in determining the number of representatives from that district (though of course the slaves themselves could not vote). Jefferson made this a condition of the South entering the Union. The issue festered until the Civil War shattered the whole.

Any genius disturbs everyday consensual reality. Very probably, any genius experiences some anxiety for the way he or she is thrown out of step with the corporate group—without which one cannot live. Jefferson was and remained an artist-thinker. He stamped Monticello with his mythic involvements and daydreams. One of Jefferson's favorite preoccupations—and, I think, antidotes for his anxiety—was the study of Greek and Roman architecture. When he built such structures they were, in effect, outer bodies that more or less contained and modulated his opposing impulses and fevers. They were iconic paradigms of order. Even the details of the plaster cornice-work of Monticello were rich with pagan embellishments. A garlanded bull looks out at us as it is led to be sacrificed. Other panels depict tutelary spirits, familiars—Emerson called these auxiliaries, helpers. Jefferson took minute care of the estate's gardens, planning the varieties of flowers so that they bloomed in unbroken sequence through the summer season. As an old man of eighty, his exercise was limited for the most part to taking a few turns around the garden. It's nice to think that he could still find himself entranced by the beauty of the earth.

The Founders were like jugglers trying to learn new tricks; or, more playfully put, they were trying to compose a fugue of immense proportions encompassing a great variety of themes. How to keep in play individual ego, region, nation, pride, idealism, greed, fear—and all without a king to act as big boss? The Founders were making up a nation as they went along. It is no accident that the radically improvisational and experimental music called jazz emerged in the United States. As we all know, the first stage of the experiment exploded in a massive civil war seventy-five years later.

Plato described the statesman as one who somehow balances incommensurables, who somehow compares apples and oranges; we may suggest, anachronistically, one who engages in a somewhat *atonal* world. Seen in these terms, the Civil War indicated a widespread and catastrophic failure of statesmanship. The jugglers had dropped their objects, the fugue had unraveled. But all these metaphors suffice only so far. Jugglers, after all, have a limited number of things to juggle—knives, Indian-pins, tennis balls, whatever—and they juggle onstage in protected situations. But in everyday life, life in the raw, the influences that work on each of us every instant are not isolable and enumerable. The context of life is the much-at-once, and we can't get it all in front of us, numbered, objectified, managed; we ourselves are part of what is being juggled and drawn into its matrix.

I have fashioned yet another metaphor: strands to be woven. But this has limitations as well, for it suggests a process that is much more deliberate and under our control than is the case in actual life. Most of what we commonly call weaving is highly deliberate; the patterns to be woven are planned, envisioned ends-in-view. Moreover, we have mastered the means to achieve these ends. Other kinds of weaving—or "weaving" understood metaphorically—seem quite accidental. It is more as if things or persons by happenstance *become woven* into others. Hairs fall from the head and insinuate themselves into woven clothing, straws in the wind entangle themselves in boluses of materials already started and augment them, animals may burrow into them and find warmth in winter to survive.

Above all, these reflections reignite our realization of what we don't know that we don't know. This is the lure that will energize us if we only stay open to it—for we are hunters still. This is what will rescue us from the emotional emptiness and flatness of the totally secularized and routinized life. Emerson noted that the secret of living is to live by abandonment. That is, the abandonment of constant calculation, allowing spontaneity. These geniuses might perhaps be contagious presences for us.

Our experimental nation is now at the forefront of the world, for better or for worse. The next genius to whom I turn in the attempt to grasp what is happening so rapidly in our era is the American philosopher-scientist Charles Sanders Peirce. He contributed mightily to what has come to be called the pragmatic tradition of thought, but he and the tradition have been greatly misunderstood because our culture projects its presumptions of control, mastery, and "practicality" on whatever it thinks about. The culture mindlessly projects the dominance of vision—the distancing and objectifying sense par excellence.

Peirce had a deep appreciation of what, following William James, I have called the much-at-once. For him, voluntary inquiry and deliberate thinking never start from scratch—from a clean slate. Rather, it starts within an inherited mass or bolus that cannot be inventoried: Following the insight of one of Peirce's mentors, F. W. J. Schelling, it is *unprethinkable*. Before we find anything, and begin to articulate what we have found, we have already been found by the world, already deeply influenced, molded, tuned. To repeat just one of the more obvious things: Before any of us can use the pronoun *I*, we have already been found, named. Before I can say *I*, we must have heard *my call*. A later "pragmatist" John Dewey makes the point in his own way. For any inquiry of any sort to get underway, it must start within the felt qualities, the qualia, of the whole encompassing situation. To free our inquiries of unwitting constrictions we must become at least semi-adequately aware of these encompassing and interfusing qualia. When we do, we realize that we have always already been *attuned* by and to the world in one way or another.

One polar opposition that William James found to be actually helpful was thick/thin. If we would hope to grasp our actual reality, we must *thicken up* our descriptions of where we already stand—or stumble—within the much-at-once. We must not become entranced with neat, compact, harmonious sets of abstractions, but feel our way into the density of the much-at-once. We must learn to love concreteness and adequacy as we learn how to live. In fact, learning to live is learning to find our own music. The music of Henry Bugbee's prose makes this point, especially when intoned ritualistically:

> As true stillness comes upon us, we hear, we hear, and we learn that our whole lives may have the character of finding that anthem which would be native to our own tongue, and which alone can be the true answer for each of us to the questioning, the calling, the demand for ultimate reckoning which devolves upon us. (*The Inward Morning: A Philosophical Exploration in Journal Form*, 221)

If we take our cue from Kant, we will think that genius is the ability to invent rules when the old ones suffocate growth. So, too, the Founders improvised. They realized that people are naturally absorbed in special interests and by monocular vision. People only resonate with what they happen to be tuned into at the time. In trying to assess the intrabodily "psychical" costs of the tensions activating geniuses, it helps to compare Jefferson to Peirce, born thirteen years after Jefferson's death in 1826. Both would lose weeks and months of their lives to ferocious migraine headaches. As we've noted, after employing his poetic genius to write the Declaration of Independence—whole days running together—Jefferson was incapacitated for weeks.

Considering Peirce's tensions, he was so innovative and idiosyncratic, so in advance of most of the best academic-philosophical thinkers of the time, that he could not gain lasting employment in a university philosophy department, but could make a living only outside academia as a scientist and mathematician. With granitic integrity, he tried for a lifetime to connect his science with his broad interpretive vision. It was the vision of a living, evolving cosmos, of our role within it as feeling, thinking, revering, intertwining, and ancient and growing organisms. Peirce was a scientist who was also moved by the depth of myth and the twilight zone of dreaming—what he called *musing*.

Peirce claimed that his first memory was of himself at the age of four hearing Emerson talk about Nature. This remained a lifelong major influence. We can't hope to speak for a transcendent God, nor even about such a being, thought Peirce, but we can hope to delve with the most attuned senses, and lovingly, into the here and now, the much-at-once, and discover all-nurturing continuities and evolvings between things. This analogizes Emerson's "inexplicable continuity of this web of God"; it is that which can be experienced only by the sensorium and the heart perceiving in the closest tandem. To think that we can detach ourselves from the much-at-once and, like a transcendent God, achieve perfect factual objectivity—to think that we can stand above history and grasp it comprehensively—is to play at being a Transcendent Being oneself. It is to misunderstand from the start our actual situatedness. We are in the much-at-once, in over our heads. To claim to take the God's-eye point of view is incredibly presumptuous and dangerous.

No matter how merely factual and detached our perceptions and judgments may seem to be, *apparently,* we are always already involved emotionally in some way to some extent. Anything whatsoever that we notice must be of at least minimal interest and value to us: "The fly is on the table." "These are wads of gum deposited on the sidewalk long ago." We are not pure intellects that happen to be attached for a while to a body, but are thinking animals seeking to adapt and survive within a Nature that never lets us go—no matter how hard we try to insulate ourselves in inventions and artificial environments. We can only delve, innovate, explore, experiment, then delve, innovate, explore, and experiment some more.

Peirce's whole encompassing vision could only be experimental. The real explorer cannot rely on old routes, classifications, maps, segregations, inclusions, exclusions. Distinctions that work well enough in a settled culture and in times of low stress can fatally impede or block growth in a culture that has cut itself loose from many of its traditions and comforts, venturing into unknown seas with ever greater acceleration. What was not doubtful for our hunter-gatherer forebears, since their survival depended on high experiential probability, may become doubtful for a culture caught up in ever-changing science and technology. But long-ingrained verbal habits remain. It is so easy to *say* that A is not B, and practices quickly aggregate around the distinctions drawn, that this ease blinds us to our own oversimplified exclusions, leading to the inevitable constrictions and hardenings of our experience. Facile binary oppositions typically enthrall, and not for the better. If something is not A, it must be B, and if not B, then A. For example, if something is no longer present, it must be past. But if we attend closely to what actually occurs in experience, something may not be occurring exactly now, but as it recedes in time it retains a sort of presence that weaves itself through our experiencing fugally, contrapuntally, and sustainingly; the metaphor of the fugue, again, proves helpful.

The constricting and impoverishing oppositions seem endless. If some organism, say, is not biologically female, it must be male, and vice versa. But if we attend closely to what actually turns up in experience, we find that some organisms denominated female behave more like the average male does; and likewise some males with respect to the average female. We must sort things out to have a world in experience, but our ways of sorting easily petrify our attention when we should be supple, balanced, alert, innovative. We actually live in vagueness and in blurry borderlands. People with a tendency to pigeonhole and categorize were uncomfortable with Peirce, and since he had to live with them, he had to experience considerable discomfort of his own. So creative was he that people tended to think of him—as many had thought of Jefferson—as unstable.

The most crippling binary opposition is the one between mind and matter, or soul and body. The so-called father of modern philosophy, René Descartes, had most deeply drawn this distinction, and Peirce believed that the first business of our era was to jettison Cartesianism. For believing in the mind/matter dualism, we are divorced within ourselves and divorced from the rest of Nature as well. Thus detached, we think we look at a world "out there" from which all deep kinship vanishes, and if things attract us it is only as objects to be dominated and exploited. "Mind" is a mere word parading as a thing or a domain, and the reification of the word engenders a crippling binary opposition: either "in the mind" or outside of it. But when alert to our actual experiencing, we realize that all awareness, though it may have a focus, shades off on all sides into the margins, the fringes, the vague, and blurs into the surround—the world-experienced, where instinct tells us we should be at home. The polar opposition of mind and matter blocks the weaving of the strands of our lives, whether the weaving is voluntary or not.

For Peirce there is no reason we can give for being reasonable, for if we try to give a reason, we are already being reasonable. To be reasonable is a kind of primal choice that we must make and remake. Moreover, there is no one way that the truly creative are choosing, but there are as many ways to be reasonable as may prove fruitful in different contexts of need, desire, experience, as may navigate us successfully through the encompassing and never perfectly transparent world. In one of his first essays, Peirce wrote:

> Philosophy ought to imitate the successful sciences in its methods, so far as to proceed only from tangible premises which can be subjected to careful scrutiny, and to trust rather to the multitude and variety of its arguments than to the conclusiveness of any one. His [the philosopher's] reasoning should not form a chain which is no stronger than its weakest link, but a cable whose fibres may be ever so slender, provided they are sufficiently numerous and intimately connected. ("Some Consequences of Four Incapacities," in *Collected Papers of Charles Sanders Peirce*, 5:157)

Weaving together multitudes of slender strands! What sort of metaphor is that? Just visual? Or also tactile, kinesthetic, musical, as we remember how primal peoples weave nets and baskets from strands of fiber they have created by rubbing together stems of flax or blades of grasses between their hands or against their thighs, and that melodies are made of interweaving lines of notes and rhythmic beats.

To allude yet again to one of the memorable phrases of Peirce's friend and helpmeet William James: The world is the "much-at-once," indefinitely variegated, changing, voluminous, overflowing all our categories and classifications. It owns us and places us before we can own and place anything else. If we are alert, we realize that there are more sorts of things going on all around and through us than we can imagine looking for. It is blind arrogance to think we can begin with a few self-evident truths or axioms, from which all else can be deduced with necessity. We constantly undergo an oceanic world of many pulses and currents: We are sunk in it over our heads. Again, James:

> Music gives us ontological messages which non-musical criticism is unable to contradict, though it may laugh at our foolishness in minding them. There is a verge of the mind which these things haunt; and whispers therefrom mingle with the operations of our understanding, even as the waters of the infinite ocean send their waves to break among the pebbles that lie upon our shores. (*The Varieties of Religious Experience*, lecture 9, 334)

To claim to be an atom isolated from everything else is presumptuous and dangerous. Whether we acknowledge it or not, we are always already involved in humanity *and* animality. If we find ourselves at all, we find ourselves already shaped by others, by other living and nonliving things. These are not just general or abstract ideas "in the mind," not mere "universals seen by the eye of the mind." Indicated in the words *humanity* and *animality* are general tendencies to act and be together in certain ways in the cosmos. In an important and difficult sense, the universe is alive.[3]

3. Peirce's attack on atomism and mechanism and his contextualism and holism are revealed in his remarks about attempts to locate thinking: "The psychologists undertake to locate various mental powers in the brain, and above all consider it as quite certain that the faculty of language resides in a certain lobe; but I believe it comes decidedly nearer the truth (though not really true)

Hence Peirce agrees with Emerson that individuals caught up in their specialties must at special times return and embrace each other in their shared humanity—at least if they would be fulfilled individuals. In an age of disruption and revolution on every hand, we must become morally and spiritually self-regulating beings. The divine is not far to seek, but—adapting a line from Augustine—it is more inward than our inmost.

Peirce was idiosyncratic (some would say antisocial) and far ahead of most other philosophers of his time; he was both a theoretician of the highest and most creative caliber and a master of the concrete. That is, he was a genius in the strict sense of someone who devises and divines his own rules. In fact, the theoretical and the concrete are inseparably interlinked in his work. The meaning of anything is *at least* what it leads us to expect for our actual experience as organisms in the much-at-once and how it opens us up to encountering that reality. The meaning of *electron*, say, is what it leads us to expect for our experience in the laboratory using our instruments and experimental apparatuses, allowing us to see our results as the manifestation of the electron. Or, to say that an act or attitude is *good* is to say that we expect fulfillment or vitality for human beings in the long run who behave this way, and that in envisioning this good we help open the way for its appearance. This is the meaning of *pragmatism,* not the often-espoused misinterpretation that it espouses "the practical."

This theoretician, being a master of the concrete as well, knew that the bright light of theory should not forever lure us down a tunnel of its own projection. We must allow ourselves at crucial times to be led by instinct. Again, he called this *musement:* allowing the free association of ideas, im-

that language resides in the tongue. In my opinion, it is much more true that the thoughts of a living writer are in any printed copy of his book than they are in his brain." Quoted from Peirce's *Collected Works* (7:364) in Halton, "Peircian Animism and the End of Civilization"; this is an indispensable article. Note also this quote from Peirce's *Collected Works*: "When we gaze upon the multifariousness of nature we are looking straight into the face of a living spontaneity. A day's ramble in the country ought to bring that home to us" (6:553). Moreover, "every true universal, every continuum, is a living and conscious being" (quoted in Halton, 140). Most academics would shy away from this radical thought—calling it animism—but it helps us to discover how much under the influence of Emerson Peirce actually was, and also to realize how relevant Peirce is to reconstructing our alienated culture, to restoring beneficial enchantment.

pulses, hunches, a kind of playing, allowing ourselves to be possessed by the muses, as the ancient Greeks understood it. Hypothesis formation, Peirce ventured, is a development of the animal's ability to guess—to imaginatively foresee what probably lies around the corner or over the hill. We allow ourselves to fall into a kind of vibrating and hyperalert trance. Amazingly, though Peirce contributed in major ways to the development of mathematical logic, he distinguished that highly focused and rigorous theoretical activity from what should be called benevolent trance-work. Mathematical logic must admit of being written down and each step of the argument checked for validity—that is, validity of structural form alone. He classified this precisely as *argumentation.*

But what he called *argument* is informal. It occurs when we are led by steps or stages or pulses that feel fitting and right overall, but for which there is no formal criterion of rightness. For example, in Peirce's "A Neglected Argument for the Existence of God" (*Collected* Papers, vol. 6), he argues that we can, in a certain "frame of mind" or attunement, directly confirm the following in our experience: that loving connections to things lead to fulfillment of human existence. Moreover, we can confirm that more is at work (or at play) than we are personally responsible for. This, Peirce proposed, must be just what we mean by *God.*

So how did Peirce hold all this together over a long lifetime of adversity? Forever pressing out the envelope into unknown territory, he paid a tremendous price. Like Jefferson, he not only suffered from migraines but was encumbered by "tangling vines and self-reproach" and castigated himself for "waste of time." Also, most chillingly, by the opposition and incomprehension of "educated society." Peirce held his work together ecstatically. I suppose that this was his way of experiencing God. He was ecstatically caught up in a self-evolving and mysterious cosmos, while most of the rest of humanity is locked into the wish-fulfilling fantasies of the child, and yet failing to encompass the child within their larger growing selves.

However self-enclosed we may seem to be, there is always this possibility that the much-at-once or our animality attuned to the larger cosmos might break through our distracted and alienated trance state. A striking instance of how, in a split second, a sudden crescendo might reach us is exhibited in the story of Kevin Hines, a young man who jumped from the Golden Gate Bridge and somehow survived (*The Bridge* [2006], a documentary film directed and produced by Eric Steel). He recounted the moments preceding his decision to kill himself. A woman passing on the walkway had asked him to take a photo of her, apparently not noticing the tears on his face—or not caring—"caught up in her own hype." This was the kind of self-absorbed trance world that had driven him to this point. Instantly after jumping, however, he realized he wanted to live. Something broke through. Some other melody of earth and life reached him, even in the midst of his plunge into extinction. He was able to adjust his falling body enough as he plummeted to strike the water feet first—and he survived.

SEGMENT SIX

THE UNITED STATES: EXPERIMENTAL NATION

We dealt with extraordinary persons in the preceding Segment 5, geniuses who were aware that they lived in a revolutionary, disrupted age, and that the United States itself was a kind of experiment. As Lincoln expressed it at Gettysburg, the venture was to see if a government of the people, by the people, for the people could long endure. We have also been dealing so far with an elite, as the mass of Americans were not aware of their existence—with the exception of Jefferson—nor were they aware of the issues with which they grappled: political, religious, ethical, mythic, cosmological. The mass of Americans were absorbed in the daily tasks of putting food on the table, avoiding another bloody confrontation with Native Americans, preventing a child from getting lost or dying, and so on. They could not imagine trying to trace Emerson's "inexplicable continuity of this web of God," his immanent divinity. If they were religious, they usually held to the simplest sort of transcendent deity, avoiding the deeper waters of complexity implied in Emerson's web of God.

Astutely, Harold Bloom writes in *The American Religion: The Emergence of the Post-Christian Nation*: "No Western nation is as religion-soaked as ours, where nine out of ten of us love God and are loved by him in return. That mutual passion centers our society and demands some understanding, if our doom-eager society is to be understood at all" (30). The first *other* for nearly all of us is another human being, typically a parent. Almost all people live locked into this relationship's impact upon our lives without being able to trace out all of its strands of interconnection. Emerson and Peirce surely had these personal bafflements, but they were also caught up ecstatically in the whole cosmos—in evolving states of hyperawareness. Even for Jefferson, "Nature and Nature's God" was no mere rhetorical formula; it somehow entranced him and he wanted to stamp the world with his understanding of it. Today it seems much of spirituality and religion have become polarized between, on the one hand, too simple a belief in fundamentalist or fideist religion that broaches no healthy doubt (doubt that is acknowledged by most theologians as essential to faith), and on the other hand, an easy secularism enmeshed with the materialistic surface of life, deaf to its deeper rhythms. The strands of fundamentalists' lives get woven together day by day, their faith continually reinforced by ritualistically repeated observances within the consensual community of fellow believers. They are entranced, but within a domain that is in fact very narrow, I believe. These observances are coordinated with the pivotal seasons of the sacred calendar and also with pivotal transitions in each believer's life: baptism, confirmation, marriage, death. The validity of these observances is attested by the authority of the church, which traces this authority to a divine origin. Secular intellectuals are often unable to grasp the existential potency and gravity of these religious practices, and the nation is now as splintered into subcultures as at any time since the Civil War.

The existential philosopher Gabriel Marcel writes of the "broken world"—that is, a technocratic world in which any sense of wonder concerning the ontological is silenced by an unconscious relativism or by a monism that discounts the personal, ignores the tragic, and denies the transcendent (*The Philosophy of Existentialism*, 15). The barren fate of many Americans today is to believe no longer in such a transcendent Father figure, or the rituals that afford access to him and to his care. Hence their fate is to live bereft of belief in *anything* sacred. This too often means a flat and empty life and/or the frantic pursuit of distractions and the crudest pleasures—not to mention addictions.

The founding fathers of the United States gave expression to an experimental nation that sought to ask: Without benefit of overriding authorities such as popes and kings, can we govern ourselves sanely? Can we govern through reasoning and dialogue and by principles we consider reasonable? As we all know, the experiment went into convulsions about eighty years later in the monstrous Civil War. The questions are far from rhetorical. No sure answers to them are yet available. Our distinctively human use of symbols and signs allows us to dream up utopias, to dream up "spirits," "substances," and "entities" of the most questionable sorts. Take, for example, the "mind"—commonly and disastrously equated with consciousness. Following the modernism of Descartes, mind is supposed to be a kind of shadowy entity that has mental "contents," and is assumed to have the reflective power to inventory those contents. In reality, however, what is verifiable is that we are vulnerable organisms that, on occasion, think, perceive, misperceive, attend, selectively inattend, dream, hallucinate, are at times possessed by emotions like despair and rage, are bored, and so on. We have powers of self-deception, individual and corporate, and the ability to mask out truths that boggle the "rational mind." Artists of many kinds exhibit this to our appalled regard, as do psychoanalysts and quite a few scientists.

The Constitution of the United States, the founding document of this experimental nation, displays the ominous mischievousness of the human "mind." A crucial example: The document never uses the term "slavery" but only sneakily acknowledges it in euphemisms and declares that the slave trade will become illegal in 1800. General Charles Pinckney, representative of South Carolina, saw to it that this was postponed until 1808. Slave trade was de jure punishable by death, but the law was not enforced until President Lincoln did so in a highly controversial case during the Civil War many decades later. The number of slaves grew to about four million. Lincoln, speaking of the Constitution and its less than straightforward treatment of slavery, declared in 1854:

> Thus the thing is hid away . . . just as an afflicted man hides away a wen or a cancer, which he dares not cut out at once, lest he bleed to death; with the promise, nevertheless, that the cutting may begin at the end of a given time. . . . They hedged and hemmed it into the narrowest limits of necessity. (William Lee Miller, *President Lincoln: The Duty of a Statesman*, 238)

The cunning duplicity of which the human "mind" is capable is attested to in the observation of Don Fehrenbacher: "It is as though the Framers were half-consciously trying to frame two constitutions, one for their own time and the other for the ages, with slavery viewed bifocally—that is, plainly visible at their feet, but disappearing as they lifted their eyes" (quoted in Miller, *President Lincoln*, 239). Talk about split consciousness! But it is not Descartes's so-called "mental substance" that is split. Rather, it is awareness generated by a vulnerable, unstable, frightened, self-congratulating animal-organism called human. To be split in awareness means that some things are done with no conscious awareness, or as I have expressed it, in a trance. Somehow, even in the most exalted circles of reason at the time, African human beings could be perceived as not fully human. The institution of slavery was a staple of Southern agricultural society, and existed as well in the North, so that for hundreds of years in our experimental nation, an experiment in freedom, there existed a canker of contradiction: the obscene institution in which humans enslave fellow human beings, and yet the contradiction was not obvious to many.

Hundreds of thousands or millions of slaves toiled in the fields, factories, and homes in the United States—each one three-fifths of a human being for legal and political purposes, but in most cases much less than that in the broader society. One can say of their background that it was very nearly wiped out. Torn from various areas and nations of the huge continent of Africa, their roots and their communities were systematically attacked or eroded by slave traders and owners. Families in formation would usually be disbanded in order to make them satellites of the slave owner's family. To take orders, they had to learn Pidgin English.

As stressed in Part I, the structure of selves and social groups is fugue-like. The very continuity of the self through time requires that events just past be retained and allowed to have their own presence, in however foggy and marginal ways. When the capacity of immediate consciousness is exceeded, "muscle memory"—as Russian stage director Constantin Stanislavski put it—holds the past in some shape, as does long-term memory in the nervous system, as recollection. The identity of the group through time requires that it confirm its members' recollections. Recollection supplies the group with stories, legends, memorials, rites, and rituals tied typically to cardinal milestones in the cycle of the year, maybe to a jubilee year such as the fiftieth or seventy-fifth. The group typically glorifies and canonizes its own past. This is at least as integral to the group and its members' reality as what actually happened at the time—insofar as this is ever knowable. Without such appropriation of its own past in its own places, the group lacks an identity, lacks reality, and likewise lacking are members' individual identities—so essentially social and cultural are we mimetically engulfed, conditioned organisms.

A slaveholder himself, Jefferson and his thought haunt our collective memory: *We hold these truths to be self-evident, that all men are created equal, that they are endowed by their Creator with certain unalienable Rights, that among these are Life, Liberty and the pursuit of Happiness.* Slaves had been deprived of their own most essential right: liberty; the freedom to move on the earth as self-moving organisms, prompted by need or desire. Slaves had been stripped nearly totally of whatever African past might have been retrieved, recapitulated—that which could have empowered, guided, woven them, one and all, out of the past and into a future. They had to, and did, radically improvise. Under these privative conditions, slaves and former slaves brewed their own language. What is called the Gullah dialect, or creole—a mixture of African, French, English, and other elements. This new intersubjectivity and intercorporeality was a new power. Speakers just born in their speaking empowered each other; they confirmed each other in their perceptions, memories, plans. They had a chance to tell their side of the story, or quite a different story altogether.

As Hegel observed two centuries ago, if slaves are to survive, they must develop certain great strengths. Like Black Elk and his people on the harsh plains of the north-central United States, they must learn endurance to the extent that their learning structures their whole body-selves, structures every breath they take, every beat of their hearts. Can one get to the next breath, the next beat? They had to create a present; they had to create a past to be appropriated as their own. They were winnowed down to essentials. To survive, African-American slaves had, as it were, to reinvent human life. Subjected to the practices of Christianity, they had to appropriate the Hebrew-Christian stories and make them their own. *They* were the slaves laboring under the cruel Egyptian Pharaoh, who had to create a present so throbbing and powerful that it supplied the material for a past and future; *they* must be delivered from their masters *someday*. Using the template of biblical stories, they created and recreated, wove and rewove their own story of deliverance from enslavement. They developed their own distinctive Christian assemblies, ecstatic antiphonals between pastors and congregants, total conversations, ecstatic participations, oral and dance traditions, fired by animistic energies, grafting these unabashedly onto Hebrew-Christian traditions. These assemblies can be understood only in religious-artistic terms, particularly those of music and dance; a parallel to the goat-man chorus in early Greek theater is not overdrawn.

American slaves made do with the little they had: gourds converted into handmade rattles; combs covered by stretched wax paper into which they blew and created music; whistles made of grass stems pulled between pressed-together thumbs; and animal skins pulled over discarded wheels or kegs employed as drums. (Slaveholders in the United States typically banned drums, fearing slaves would communicate and plot rebellion, but with one interesting exception: drumming was allowed on Sunday afternoons in Congo Square in New Orleans; elsewhere, great African traditions of drumming were carried on, mainly in Cuba and Brazil.) The most important instrument of all was the body, made percussive and catapulted into communal dance, chant, clapping, stamping, song. It was as if this segment of the human race had to reinvent itself in a situation of abject privation. Propulsive music was essential to survival, as essential as the next breath, the next beat of the heart. It is one thing to listen in one's armchair to a kinetic Beethoven symphony or fugue. It is another to sing and dance and percuss with one's body because one's life depends on it. Clapping and stomping is percussing; the essentials are the same.

Slaves were turned to the essentials: gasping for the next breath, prizing the next beat of the heart, experiencing inexpressible gratitude that one's child was still alive. Those who survived gained great strength. Pearl S. Buck draws a portrait of creative people as organisms in extremis:

> The truly creative mind in any field is no more than this: A human creature born abnormally, inhumanely sensitive. To them a touch is a blow, a sound is a noise, a misfortune is a tragedy, a joy is an ecstasy, a friend is a lover, a lover is a god, and failure is death. Add to this cruelly delicate organism the overpowering necessity to create, create, create—so that without the creating of music or poetry or books or buildings or something of meaning, their very breath is cut off. (Quoted in Diane Ackerman, *An Alchemy of Mind: The Marvel and Mystery of the Brain*, 159)

This immense improvisation by African Americans occurred within a nation of states, actual and potential, also improvising its own creation. Most enslaved peoples through the ages have left very few records. One is tempted to say that they and their works are made to simply vanish. But this is not true of African-American slaves. Many of their creations have been caught up, alive and tingling, in our evolving life. The slaves' music, which provided the roots for jazz, transformed the nation and its ways of being musically expressive. When conventional instruments were obtained along with freedom, what became Dixieland jazz was born. A troupe of musicians would play a dirge after a funeral on the way to the graveyard, then on the way home after the service of interment they would play their incredibly upbeat, sparkling jazz. Thus the ever-regenerating universe is signaled, recovering within itself and going on, circular power returning into itself. Once again, this stratum of shared existence, defining who we are together, is, in Emerson's words, the seamless continuity of the web of God.

Human reality must include the stories that we tell about ourselves repeatedly. The stories are as much sung as told, as early storytellers, the bards, accompanied themselves with small harps, say. These stories are selections from our past that are created, retrieved, appropriated and reappropriated, with rough edges rounded off and facets and connections polished and developed through reiteration. It is not enough for us to do things and then report the bare facts: We ate the evening meal; we went to the funeral; we watched the sun come up; we engaged in coitus. We must interpret these events, reinterpret them, interpret the interpretations, and perhaps contest others' interpretations. Biologically speaking, we are primates, but ones blessed (or cursed?) with the endless elaborative powers of human speech and art. The reality we live is a semisolid, quivering bolus of fact and fiction, actual event and fantasy, with the one merging imperceptibly and constantly into the other. We are creatures both of our circumstances and of the evolving myths that we weave around us, and in which we are caught up. Certain excesses of these powers stand out, so inevitable and typical are they: Perhaps we can call them natural excesses, natural ecstasies; we naturally overflow ourselves (see Alphonso Lingis, *Excesses: Eros and Culture*). Prominent is the de facto deification of one's homeland and history. This is at least as real as what might be disclosed by "bare facts," assuming these even exist.

But is there one nation of the United States? I've already noted that all groups share through time one matrix, one land, however vaguely it be envisioned by the populace. There could be a corporate body because there was a shared land, a vague but profound sense of the mass and physiognomy of this shared land. The whole country was experimental, growing this way and that, including geographically. New lands acquired—much here, a little there—the shared land was being shaped into a fuller and more comely physiognomy in the eyes of those whose project was to build a nation, a bodily-corporate meaning. However, shared land is a necessary but not a sufficient condition of nationhood.

For the Euro-American thinkers I have stressed, and for most people of their ethnicity, something very new was occurring in the New World: a new creativity. But for Native Americans following this current, it would not be new to them (see John Neihardt, *Black Elk Speaks: Being the Life Story of a Holy Man of the Oglala Sioux*). They had never ceased to experience through their whole body-selves a kinship with Nature all around and through them, taking aspects of the land deeply into their sense of themselves. It was repeatedly memorialized in their cycling stories, rites, rituals, sacred inscriptions, and objects. The two-leggeds belong with the four-leggeds and the flying, crawling, hopping, slithering ones. They felt this kinship with vegetation too: The great World Tree at the center of their experience, blooming every spring, ensconced in their legends and visions, sent its rising and falling sap and its scent into them. At the age of nine, in a coma and nearly dying, Black Elk had a vision of the "one great hoop of the world":

> Then I was standing on the highest mountain of them all, and round about beneath me was the whole hoop of the world . . . And I saw that the sacred hoop of my people was one of many hoops that made one circle, wide as daylight and as starlight, and in the center grew one mighty flowering tree to shelter all the children of one mother and one father. And I saw that it was holy. (Neihardt, *Black Elk Speaks*, 33)

Thus blessed, he was obliged to share his blessing with his people: to have it fed through them and back to him would be to have it confirmed, and to enact it for them all would be to have it fed back through him yet again: a never-ending confirmation of individual and communal being. This was, for them, an ever-evolving fugue—de facto eternity.

The propitious moment happens nine years later when he is told that a tribal member's sick boy desperately needs help. Preparing himself for his first opportunity to cure, Black Elk spends a cold night outside, some distance from the encampment, weeping for all unhappy things. He also sees a myriad of blurry faces of those still unborn.

> It was a clear evening with no wind, and it seemed that everything was listening hard to hear something. While I was looking over there I felt that somebody wanted to talk to me. So I stood up and began to sing the first song of my vision. (137)

Something somewhere wanted to speak with him. It is not precisely located but oceanic; it comes to him from all over the sky, from all around him and beneath him. This Encompassing Presence and glorious much-at-once dilates him and organizes him and he rises and sings the song:

> Behold! A sacred voice is calling you!
> All over the sky, a sacred voice is calling! (137)

Before anything can be picked out, found, appropriated, we have been found by the world, placed, appropriated by the world, woven into and through it. In *The Varieties of Religious Experience*, James evokes "the curious sense of the whole residual cosmos that everyone possesses," but only some at certain moments can acknowledge and articulate. John

Dewey, in *Experience and Nature,* homed in on this stabilizing and centering experience of the surrounding matrix: Each "this" picked out presupposes a "system of meanings focused at a point of stress and uncertainty" that calls out for resolution. But that system was there in germ beforehand, and when we are receptive, dilated, relaxed, it may quietly move in from all around to support, orient, and place us. We allow the world to speak to us about everything, including ourselves and how we are placed within the Whole. Our attentiveness to it allows the world to speak, to speak again and again. Primal experiencing is basically oceanic and musical. World artists are caught up in the flooding surf of the unprethinkable.

Emerson rode on the tide of indigenous sensibility that has been with humanity, very probably, from the beginnings of human evolution. We are not merely predators to variously attack things *in* the world. We ourselves are *worldly*: born out of the womb of the world-experienceable, born out of meta-amniotic fluid. We are prewoven and melded by the whole of Nature: Our signs and symbols try to capture and weave this further. Emerson held to this course even when confronted by the obdurate power and prejudice of our new nation-state in formation, a nation that was learning to be imperial in its own way. He was particularly outraged at the forced displacement of the Cherokee people from their native region to the wastes of "Indian country" in Oklahoma: the infamous march, undersigned by President Andrew Jackson, known as the Trail of Tears. This was not a mere "relocation" of people on a Cartesian grid of space but a violent rupture of ties between the embodied being of a people and the land with which it had bonded.

In Black Elk's first cure, the sick boy lies at the northeasterly point on the round tepee floor, at the intersection of the direction from which come the "winds of the North that teach endurance," and the East, the direction from which come new beginnings each day. Black Elk enters through the tepee opening, which is the East. He brings a retinue of attendants and proceeds in the direction of the South. Virgins play a crucial role, as they hold the bodily potential for new life. Drummers follow. Black Elk smokes from the pipe and offers the laden smoke to the authority of the South, the Grandfather there, the source of heat and life. Then in pulses from the drum he proceeds to the West, offering smoke to the Grandfather there: the authority of death, where the sun sets each day, and where each of us must go someday—as Black Elk had nearly done nine years earlier when being prepared for his ministerial function.

At this point in the process, the sick boy smiles at him, and Black Elk feels reassured in his first attempt at curing. With the drum "arousing the mind," he feels a strange feeling coming up through his legs from Mother Earth. He drinks from a wooden cup of water in which float flakes of red willow bark. The cup is carried by a virgin for the boy to drink also. Black Elk and his group proceed to where the boy lies. The healer stamps on the earth in pulses of four. Then he kneels, placing his mouth on the boy's abdomen and sucking the cold wind of the North, which teaches endurance, through the boy's body. After instructing a virgin to help the boy rise, he leaves the tepee in the direction of the East, from which he had first entered, without waiting to monitor events further. Neihardt relates that the boy lived until thirty (156).

What is happening in this ritual? The people and their experiential cosmos weave themselves through the boy's weakened body and hold him within this great circle, so that he doesn't fall away? Is it Emerson's "circular power returning into itself," "the inexplicable continuity of this web of God"? I think that Peirce might say that a powerful and well-grounded stream of semiosis, of signs, is fed through the sick boy's body: magnetic and arresting icons and indexes. A reductionist skeptic might claim that this is "only subjective," not concrete, not the north wind in its "objective reality," but why suppose that the "real" north wind is what it is only *minus* its cumulative effects on a people through many generations? That supposition is the abstraction, the relative unreality! Today what many people caught up in secularism and scientism call "nature" is really subnatural.

What we must stretch to grasp ecstatically is this all-involving way of participating in the interfeeding life of the cosmos (see Peirce, for example, on what he defined as *synechism*: "that tendency of philosophical thought which insists upon the idea of continuity as of prime importance in philosophy and, in particular, upon the necessity of hypotheses involving true continuity," *Collected Papers* 6:169; see also "The Law of Mind"). It is a way of living in the much-at-once in which we abandon ourselves to the life shared spontaneously with everything. Everything flows into everything else and is charged and enlivened in doing so. It is all-embracing, tremulous conviviality, like that articulated by Black Elk in his vision:

> Then the Grandfathers behind me sang another sacred song from my vision. "At the center of the earth, behold a four-legged. They have said this to me!" And as they sang, a strange thing happened. My bay pricked up his ears and raised his tail and pawed the earth, neighing long and loud to where the sun goes down. And the four black horses raised their voices, neighing long and loud, and the whites and the sorrels and the buckskins did the same; and all the other horses in the village neighed, and even those out grazing in the valley and on the hill slopes raised their heads and neighed together. Then suddenly, as I sat there looking at the cloud, I saw my vision yonder once again—the tepee built of cloud and sewed with lightning, the flaming rainbow door and, underneath, the Six Grandfathers sitting, and all the horses thronging in their quarters; and also there was I myself upon my bay before the tepee. (*Black Elk Speaks*, 129)

This vision strongly resonates with ideas found in twentieth-century quantum field physics, particularly superposition and nonlocality. Gone today are assumptions of seventeenth-century mechanistic science: matter viewed as inert and always conserved; elements as fundamentally and irreducibly individual, and the whole a mere set of elements; the world as a machine with easily locatable and substitutable parts. Alfred North Whitehead, thinking in light of the successes of relativistic and field theories in physics, and on the verge of eruptive formulations of quantum theory, wrote of the intertwined fallacies of misplaced concreteness and simple location that dog us from the past. Quantum physicist David Bohm similarly writes that certain entities that have originally been combined show a peculiar nonlocal relationship, "which can best be described as a non-causal connection of things that are far apart" (Bohm, *Wholeness and the Implicate Order*, 175). Are people who share a common origin bonded together noncausally?

For all the vastness of a generalized alienation that so many experience in our North Atlantic culture, lacking any sense of such interconnectedness and bonding, at least we can say that slavery in its most brazen form has pretty well been eliminated, at least here. Maybe we approach a bit closer to a concrete and behaviorally significant sense of our shared humanity. I say this very cautiously because the culture is so fragmented, so peddled out and spilled into drops, as Emerson says, that one wonders indeed if it can ever be gathered. Try to imagine the scale of what is to be grasped. Some observers point to the Internet as a unifying force. This is not completely absurd, but it is offset by the sheer scale of things to be grasped—and for most people, grasped *through* the Internet. The limits of the Internet conceal themselves. Identity theft, for example, is a multibillion-dollar business made possible by the Internet. Why talk of identifying with the putative nisus of humanity or of the cosmos, when fellow human beings matter not a whit to so many? Some feel it to be impossible—beyond conceivability—to identify their personal good with the good of the whole, the good of humanity and the planet. How can our "minds" comprehend or get around this floating, foggy, generalized alienation that feels normal? The Internet communicates staggering quantities of information nearly instantaneously, but can it grip us with the *presence* of persons and things? Can it grip us as Li Po is gripped by Ching-Ting Peak—that of which he never grows tired, nor it of him? Is there a cure for a never-ending staleness that undermines our very recognition of it?

Alienation is truly profound and far-reaching. Few of my students have ever directly experienced the night sky blanketed with stars. That is, they have never directly experienced the Milky Way, our own home galaxy. Signs such as "DON'T DUMP HERE—DRAINS INTO OCEAN" placed on sewers and storm drains may serve to broaden awareness. But who could imagine that the great fish of the sea, tuna and swordfish, would be tainted with poisons such as mercury? How did we drink up the sea, asked Nietzsche's madman, how did we sponge away the line of the horizon (*The Gay Science*, §125)?

Shelby Foote makes the interesting point that before the Civil War occurred, people said "These are the United States," and afterward "This is the United States" (Foote, *The Civil War*). True, perhaps, but nothing is more misleading than the truth when it is misleading. For today legions of secularized people apparently find it impossible to consort civilly with fundamentalist Christian "hinterlanders in the flyover states," and these "benighted" folks return the compliment, of course. Great numbers of citizens of the United States do not feel at home in their own country, let alone in the world at large. More is at work in this generalized alienation than just dumb incomprehension of Islam, say, or of why their fundamentalists hate us so. We Euro-Americans have disenchanted and pulverized the experienced world. Yet as James put it, there may be no hope, but if we don't hope, there's certainly none. It is reasonable to hope. And we can couple this insight with that of the poet Hölderlin: Where danger lies, there also lies deliverance ("Patmos"). The thing most to be feared, I believe, is stupor and the humdrum—the bad, relentless trance.

The American composer Charles Ives ranks with Schoenberg and his students as a master of atonal music. Through his music he discloses the immediacy of our experiencing today in a world no longer appropriable and experienceable within traditional rites, rituals, rules, set codes. What would happen if we did not preunderstand, prepackage, only selectively attend (or inattend) to our experiencing, but let our experiencing in the United States today disclose itself in its fresh amplitude and raw immediacy? This open experiencing is difficult, but Charles Ives's efforts as composer and ours as listeners are rewarding. Through the streaming much-at-once of the moment, impossible to classify, emerges fragments of patriotic or religious hymns. The self here and now retrieves and recuperates itself as past. And not only the individual self but that self caught up in the collective and the experiencing of the national group. Ives's music engages us, perhaps after an initial shock, because *ourselves* in our immediacy engage us, and as I've been questioning all along, what could engage us more?

All over in European art and music of the nineteenth and twentieth centuries a deeply nostalgic turn was being taken. We saw it at work in Shostakovich's last works, indicated in his fascination with folk music, particularly Jewish. Bela Bartok, for one, made a systematic study of Hungarian folk songs. We should refer also to Bedrich Smetana and Antonin Dvořák, among others. This reflected the widespread conviction that change was occurring too rapidly all over the world. If selves and group-selves are not simply to fly to pieces, their pasts must be methodically retrieved and reappropriated, regathered, made newly our own. We must somehow create an enthralling fugue of gargantuan proportions.

But there is something unique about Ives. Evident is the peculiarly improvisatory, precarious, poignant, and down-home quality of the New World that held him, within which he composed. Our hearing of his music, knowing that it was greatly unappreciated by his countrymen at the time, only adds to the poignancy and precariousness of the experience. Ives was disclosing more about us than most of us, his contemporaries, could bear to face and acknowledge. When Ives composes atonally on the theme of the death of Lincoln and we suddenly hear strains of the traditional Christian hymn, *Nearer My God to Thee*, we are found through our past immediately, directly, concretely. But reassuringly? Some at least are imbued with the solidity and buoyancy of song, and we might recall that Black Elk, interrogated on the heath by *something* that wanted to speak to him, replied by rising and singing the song from his great vision.

When I hear these sudden strains emerge from Ives, I experience the buoyancy of the music in my bodily self—in my bony, ligamented, earth-planted, blood-coursing self—but it's a buoyancy that is painfully nostalgic, that cannot be held solidly in my grip:

> There is a fountain filled with blood
> Drawn from Emmanuel's veins
> And sinners plunged beneath that flood
> Lose all their guilt and stains.

Ives speaks and sings for the United States, and we might even now experience and locate ourselves through his music. We might experience a *moving* much-at-once, a multitude of diverging strands that nevertheless somehow forms a strange whole? Sometimes the rhythms and melodies from different choirs or sectors of the orchestra are so jagged and crosscutting that several conductors must be entrusted with shepherding the composition home; consider, for example, his great Fourth Symphony, composed between the years 1910 and 1916. This in itself can be a homecoming experience for a nation making itself up as it goes along, an experimental nation of incredible diversity, changing so rapidly and enduring the stresses of that.

Ives's religious or patriotic fragments are tossed up out of atonal dreams, both pleasant ones and nightmares. The music is just as shocking and nostalgic as is some late Shostakovich, but it comes with a distinctly American loose-jointedness and garb. The fragmentation might be construed this way: It tends to break the hold of a deified past, while not simply ignoring or debunking it. At the very least, Ives's treatment keeps the past alive as an issue. The past is no longer cemented prejudice or mere complacency. Even shared *questioning* is something shared—a kind of bond that might keep us together as a nation in times of grave troubles and disruptions?

It may be that a tipping point will be reached, a time when enough people have grown articulately aware of generalized alienation to try to do something about it. It just might happen that people will become sufficiently troubled by our genocide of Native Americans that we attend to them—actually for the first time—giving attention to these indigenous people, seeking to understand their past. If we do, we will discern a profound connection between them and our most prescient Euro-American thinkers earlier detailed. Might we feel at home again in Nature? As John Dewey tried to advise us, through our many-armed technological culture we radically alter Nature—but always *within* Nature. There are always consequences of what we do beyond what we can imagine, engulfed as we are in any momentary much-at-once. We might be put in touch with the outback of the universe: behind the beyond?

We certainly need to hear all that historians can tell us about how we got to our present pass. But it is not sufficient for real liberation from cemented assumptions and prejudices—the prejudicial domain of the prereflective. The dominant culture is hobbled by the unwitting assumption that facts are just "out there" awaiting detection by the detached, objectifying inquirer's scrutiny. In the process of objectifying the world, however, we automatically and immediately take leave of our own prereflective, often trance-animated experiencing within the much-at-once of any moment. So we tend not to see these prereflective workings in the persons and groups we are studying. This is the fruit of scientism: the ideology that *only* science can know reality. This is not a position supportable by science. It is an ideology.

To be unaware of the trance level is to miss a necessary condition for grasping how people behave and respond to the world, for it reaches into the magical and mythical level of experiencing. Only a few of the most attuned, perceptive, and daring thinkers penetrate to this lived level and disclose it. One of these is Jean-Paul Sartre. Take his phenomenology of fainting, for example (see *Sketch for a Theory of the Emotions*). When terrified by the abrupt appearance before us of a wild beast, say, or of a suicide bomber about detonate his explosives—what may we do? Sartre says that we may in that instant magically confuse our *awareness* of the thing with the *thing*, so that in expunging the awareness we expunge the thing—all delusionally and magically, of course. We faint.

As Sartre acknowledges in the next section of his *Sketch for a Theory of the Emotions*, however, there is a second way to understand the "magic" of emotions in prereflective experience. Although sometimes our immediate emotional response may substitute our awareness of the things in front of us for a wish to be rid of obstacles "magically," our emotions also open us to a truly magical dimension of the world in another way: to the way other beings "move us" even though they are "acting at a distance"—that is to say, with no rational or causal reasons or intermediaries. This aspect of our emotional life can connect us nonlogically with elements of the world, affirming our interrelations with seemingly foreign beings that become part of our internal reality through this interconnection. This is trance as regenerative, forging links with beings around us that amplify our own vitality and identity.

We must contend with the reality that much of the basis of human behavior is utterly irrational. When possible, we must tune into the incantatory beats that induce and animate trances of one sort or another in individuals and groups. For instance, one of the fiercest and most effective leaders in the Civil War was the Confederate cavalry general Nathan Bedford Forrest—so fierce that Union General Sherman offered a large reward for his capture, dead or alive, though the funds were never used. Forrest's tactical feats, daring, sheer physical prowess, and general deadliness sometimes appear to be uncanny. Sounding out the name Nathan Bedford Forrest, you will hear a trochaic trimeter: |—, |—, |—. You may hear in its beats, moreover, the terrifying inexorability of something more-than-human, the diabolical or demonic, the inexorability of fate. Try to imagine what this induced in him when he heard himself called by his full name, or repeated it soundlessly to himself.

Are there other examples? General Sherman's first name—Tecumseh—was bestowed on him by his biological parents after the famous Native American chief and warrior. When his parents soon died, his adoptive parents wanted a "more civilized" name, so they added William. Or consider the name of General Ulysses Simpson Grant—U. S. Grant. Can we assume that the repeated hammering of the initials "U.S." in his name had nothing to do with his magnificent obsession, shared with Lincoln, for preserving the union of the states at all costs? Educated society—as Emerson put it—very probably will dismiss all this as "impressionistic," "fabulistic," "unscientific," "romantic." There are forces on an irrational level, however, emotional movements that catch us up in their spell and promote the growth within us of special courage or talents. In being open to these forces and recognizing the music of names, places, and the possible immediate response to unavoidable suffering endured through its power, we are emulating Emerson's openness.

The etymology of "fact" in Latin is revealing. It comes from *factum*, thing done (related to "factory"). Relying on this linguistic lead, "fact" means what is concluded about the world when inquiry is thought to be done. But nearly always there is more inquiring to be done. Maybe in repeating over and over—the facts, the facts, the facts—we block the road of inquiry with bad trance. Maybe in doing so we commit what Peirce thought to be the unforgivable intellectual sin.

•

After reviewing the dangers of trance, we should not simply throw it out—or try to. Vitality requires the charms of benevolent entrancement in appropriate degrees at the appropriate junctures of life. Trance is basically a musical phenomenon, and we are musical creatures. When people are in the grip of humdrum ideological or technological trances, good music has stopped. On the eve of the nineteenth century, Friedrich Schiller wrote of the disenchantment of the world. This was a portentous and ominous observation. If we are fully alive, we will feel entranced at certain times and in certain situations; but just when and where is it so essentially enlivening?

Perhaps the most insidious aspect of technology linked with commercialism is the attempt, pounding away at us nearly all the time, to entrance us with things of limited and ephemeral value. The great values—the sacred, the holy, the numinously ecstatic—are obscured. Missing is any sense that anything is missing. For example, Bruckner's evocation of circular power returning into itself—ever recuperating, ever regenerating—is no longer heard by most. It is no longer even suspected: There are no resonances whatsoever. This power lies beyond a horizon that is not imagined. The waves of the vast ocean's surf—advancing, retreating, recuperating their power—are no longer imagined.

Following Emerson, Peirce carved out a generous domain for musement. In it we allow entrancement to occur, yet at some level or other we are aware of it *as such*. We are not engulfed in it, helpless in its grip: It is benevolent, and we are not fanatics. Flatness, vacuity, residual helplessness, and depression seem inescapable without a place and time for such benevolent entrancement. They may be escapable through it.

"Creativity" is such a nice word, and beguilingly easy to use! The actual process of profound creativity, however, can be dangerous and greatly disruptive. Genius doesn't fall down to earth from heaven readymade. It must be formed initially within the conventional mode of experiencing a world and having a world-experienced that holds for one's original, looming, surrounding, authoritative others—family, neighborhood, society, and so on. Genius must allow this conventionally experienced ground to be dislodged somewhat from beneath its feet. This does not happen only in the "head" or the "mind"; it is a disruption within the whole bodily self, as one attempts to replant oneself in a new stance on the earth. From the point of view of the conventionalized person, genius does the impossible.

With the insight of genius, James sees what is involved in the creations of genius. The actual creative process occurs on the prereflective level of immediate involvement in the world: "the instant field of the present" or the much-at-once. This is the level prior to and more fundamental than the neat distinguishing of self and other, subject and object, moving and unmoved, mind and matter—the artificial secondary stratum on which we self-deludingly believe we are in control of everything. In James's trenchant example: "When clouds float by the moon, it is as if both clouds and moon and we ourselves shared in the motion" ("The Place of Affectional Facts in a World of Pure Experience," 205). The earth itself speaks, gestures, and inspires us with flows of meaning and purpose on a prereflective, embodied level, and the rhythms of our own creativity are taken up from the much-at-once beyond the grasp of intellect.

For greatly innovative and creative people this is not merely an ephemeral and bizarre event; this sort of experience has generalized and deepened itself into a way of living off-balance for considerable stretches of time. For highly creative artists and thinkers this lack of sharp differentiation between moving body-self and other moving things figures in what John Muir called divine frenzy—the loss of balance ingredient in the excitement of true creativity. Through the genius, we partake of wilderness. The world is not made of dumb and inert matter but of movement, notes, melodies, and rhythms that sound a profound meaning within our bodies immersed in the depths of the much-at-once. We are newly and amazingly coherent responding to these beckonings.

We turn now to science as an ecstatic pursuit, often disruptive and truly amazing.

SEGMENT SEVEN

MUSIC OF SCIENCE, THOUGHT, AND THE BODY

We exist today in a titanic, planet-wide explosion of creativity and change. Elements of our lives fly off hither, thither, and yon in a crescendo of creativity, but one that threatens at times to tear itself to pieces. Can we catch our balance sufficiently even to describe it? It seems to be best conveyed in the three eruptions in Shostakovich's Fourth Symphony, or in the grinding, blaring, ear-shattering cacophonies in orchestral works by Charles Ives, George Rochberg, and Alfred Schnittke.

Each of us is sheathed in the skin of a body and we are individuated thereby, set off from other individuals (but see Appendix C on the body-schema and its role in empathy). Any uninvited penetration of this sheath—even the intimation of this possibility—is a menace and a threat. Yet this sheath is immensely porous, for it lays us open to influences from every side, real, imagined, unimagined: we are incredibly vulnerable beings within the much-at-once. As earlier noted, in our intrauterine months of life we were able to hear and feel all kinds of vibrations and sounds long before we could see anything (though there may have been some nascent visual phenomena, some synesthesia). There was the booming of sounds both from around and within the mother: the booming of her heart, the bellows of her lungs, the gurgling of her fluids, and intermixed and interwoven through all this, that responsive rapid beating of the infant's own heart. Long before each of us could use our hands to touch anything, our whole bodies responded kinesthetically to themselves in their mother's uterine environment. The fetus rode within her body, which, porous, resonated within her whole experienced-world. We floated in amniotic fluid that resonated as only that location could within the universe. Great music sometimes conveys this primal attunement and buoyancy. It can also convey the shocking jolts that must also have occurred.

Music is the furthest thing from a redundancy or superfluity. For when successful, music thematizes our primal attunements or even malattunements, establishing some breathing room between our mature reflecting selves and these primal attunements: some room for the recognition and mulling of these, and the possibility perhaps of reattunements. That is, some possibility of dislodging or unengulfing ourselves from these attunements, without necessarily losing them, some possibility of fresh air and new life. When we recognize these attunements *as* primal sorts of trances, we need not be buried alive in them if they are bad ones. We may be able to recognize bad trances *as* bad trances. Music accords us the full gift of ourselves in our actual—not merely fanciful—freedom by articulating the rhythms in which we live, allowing us to experience them more fully as revealed to our embodied selves.

Long before music can find us and free us in more or less obvious ways, we have already been found by the world. We have already been attuned one way or another. Whether in science, the arts, or whatever field of endeavor, the creative person does not prejudge or preunderstand this primal being-found but lets it work its way into his or her activity as it will, as it wriggles and turns. Even bad trances must be allowed to reveal themselves. The greatest creativity springs from the greatest letting-be and allowing. From our prenatal days the beating of the hearts, the bellows of the lungs, the gurglings of fluids and pockets of air, have found us and claimed us as ourselves—for better or worse.

The story goes that in the seventeenth century, Isaac Newton was catalyzed by the sight of a ripened apple falling "on its own" from the tree to the earth. There was no wind and no other detectable agency that could account for the fall. This happening soaked into him deeply and he searched for an explanation. He dared to hypothesize that there was some action-at-a-distance at work, what he could not precisely conceptualize, and what many of his colleagues regarded as nonsense, what we know today as the universal force of gravity. He formulated an equation to codify and accurately describe this force's workings in various circumstances, and to that extent to explain it.

But to formulate this famous law of universal gravitation, he felt forced to suppose that there was one absolute universal space and one absolute universal time. He supposed this, for they could not be experienced either with the naked senses or with the senses as extended and augmented by instruments. Within the next hundred years this was noted by Leibniz and Kant. It was not until Einstein, however, over a hundred years after Kant, that the full implications of this inability to experience absolute space and time began to appear.

Creative persons do not shrink from their vulnerability and finitude. They allow themselves to be found by the world in surprising, unpredictable, perhaps shocking ways. It seems natural to suppose that distant events take a long time for their light, their various influences, to spread and influence other events. To be open to the world, however, is to allow the possibility that distant events must occur simultaneously with closer ones—whether we can know this directly or not. Einstein questioned Newton's "natural" suppositions. He imagined that there is not one absolute time obtaining for all events: there are *times* (although this does not stop relativity physicists from trying to calculate *the* time that has elapsed since the putative big bang), and indeed, time might stop under certain very extreme conditions and circumstances.

Einstein imagined an immersion in the cycling intercirculating universe more radical and upsetting than most people dared to. He imagined an immersion in a dynamic and fluid universe that would excite in most people our ever-latent terror of abandonment or of suffocation and drowning. Outspoken and sure of his own path, Einstein was not accepted as an assistant to the great professors of physics of his time and place, so he gained no foothold of acceptance in the pyramid of academic advancement. He took a job in the patent office in Zurich, Switzerland, and kept his eyes open—or better put, he kept his whole bodily self open. One day, gazing on the clock face in a tower he imagined: What if I rode on a beam of light reflected off that clock face and kept looking at it? The appalling answer: The hands would not move, time would appear to stop.

Still locked in the assumptions of a safely compartmentalized and absolutized universe, most would say that time only *appears* to stop—it can't really stop. But Einstein was open to take as real what really appeared, to what was *given* him to think. This odd passivity, this "being found," could ground and prompt a leaping-seeking that makes possible a startling new finding. Extraordinarily creative persons are not fixated on vision and its dominance in ordinary human languages ("I see" = "I understand"). When it happens at all, seeing is just one factor in a dynamic ensemble of senses, impressions, movements, moods—a much-at-once. Recall that Einstein imagined *riding* on a beam of light reflected off the clock face. Music's great strength is that it is nonvisual—it is encompassing, kinesthetic, kinetic—not limited to ways of thinking and being cemented in our vision-dominated verbal language, our ossified and presumably detached ways of speaking and being. Music need not lead us to mindless objectifying and compartmentalizing of the world in experience. What we appropriate of the world, make our own, is a function of a dialectic of initiative and receptivity that will take an unpredictable course. Great science emerges in resonance with the piety of music (as Pythagoras knew long ago).

John Dewey, who forever distrusted all dualisms or binary oppositions, regarded science as one of the arts: specifically, the art of making mathematically precise predictions. But Dewey made a seminal distinction. Before there are "experiments in the lab," there are typically "experiments in fact" that lay a new groundwork. The play of everyday circumstances can have the power to prompt resonating attunements, impulsive or instinctive probing into previously ignored corners, crevices, horizons of the world, then waiting for what happens. This is Dewey's version of Heidegger's *Befindlichkeit*—a term that is untranslatable but roughly means, "if we find ourselves, we find ourselves already found by the world." Henry Bugbee prefers to say, in *The Inward Morning: A Philosophical Exploration in Journal Form*, that we find ourselves already *claimed* by the world. This total being in the world was memorialized by the noted contemporary physicist Richard Feynman, with a sentence left standing on his blackboard at Cal Tech upon his death: "What I cannot make I cannot understand." Making is a total activity that springs from total immersion in the fluxing world of sensuous experience, from "hands on" immediacy.

Kant had noted this many years before:

> When Galileo let balls of a particular weight, which he had determined himself, roll down an inclined plane, or Torricelli made the air carry a weight, which he had previously determined to be equal to that of a definite volume of water; or when, in later times, Stahl changed metal into lime, and lime again into metals, by withdrawing and restoring something, a new light flashed on all students of nature. They comprehended that reason has insight into that only which she herself produces on her own plan. (Second preface [1787], *Critique of Pure Reason, 2nd ed.*, in *Basic Writings of Kant*, 10)

As the pre-Socratic Greek philosopher Anaxagoras put it, we have minds because we have hands. Before Galileo and Torricelli set up their experiments, they had hunches, and these bubbled up from somewhere deep in their total bodily immersion in the world as they were immediately experiencing it. Following Emerson, Peirce knew that even the most elaborate and intricate and "far out" hypothesizing can occur only because all hypothesizing springs from a primal instinct: to guess. In order to survive, our early ancestors, including prehumans, had to be able to guess or to imagine (image) what might lie around the corner or over the hill.

Frank Waters launched his remarkable novel of the indigenous southwest, *The Man Who Killed the Deer*, with this account. A Native American is awakened at night by a message, but not in words. He hears, senses, feels attuned and claimed by this: *You are needed.* The message comes to him from the mountain behind his dwelling. Accordingly, the man saddles up his horse and both creatures are led up the mountain. They keep going up and up, with the same message sounding—or *something*—loud and clear, *You are needed.* He keeps going up with no disturbance in the message. Then at a certain point the "voice"—or whatever it is—stops altogether. This is construed by the man (and by the horse?) as his having gone far enough. He simply waits, and waits some more. Then finally in the night, very cold at that altitude, he hears a disturbance in front of him and sees dimly an injured man lying among the trees (it turns out that it is the man who killed the deer). He picks him up, straps him behind his saddle, and returns to the village.

From whence came the message that drew the man up the mountain? Why suppose a supernatural source? Isn't it more plausible to suppose that because each of us is immersed every moment in the much-at-once that each of us knows more than we *know* that we know, more than we can *reflectively acknowledge* that we know? Why not suppose that always also at work is the unencompassable domain of what we don't know that we don't know? This needn't be supernatural in the sense that it is outside Nature.

Exceptionally creative people are attuned some way within the much-at-once, and they do not turn away but attend closely to it. In the twentieth century, and now in our own, physicists are led on paths of understanding that seem baffling to common sense in this attunement. They strive for coherent accounts even when they cannot empirically confirm the things or events they are hypothesizing or postulating: for example, "strings." For about a century now there has been a disconnect in physicists' accounts of micro and macro realities, a disconnect between what is "ruled" by quantum mechanics and what by Einstein's general theory of relativity. Because of the work of Edward Whitten, there is now one unified theory of strings—incredibly small, vibrating rings—but there is no direct evidence that they exist. Quite a few physicists give them credence, nonetheless, because they connect theoretically with what *has* gained empirical confirmation. There is a deeply felt and thought, though as yet empirically unconfirmed, continuity and resonance.

Let us linger for a moment on these "strings." Research in this direction was prompted by findings concerning black holes—phenomena that result, apparently, from the implosion or collapse of large stars. What is found is the presence of something *very* small and *very* heavy. When physicists attempted to combine general relativity theory concerning the very large and heavy with the remaining three sorts of force—the strong and weak forces and electromagnetism, which concern the atomic and very small—fantastical answers emerged. An incoherence in previous theory became glaring. To create coherence, the idea of "strings" was born (and is still being born as I write). Key features of what is thought to be known about units of gravity—gravitons—were built into these postulated "entities." But then ensued a breathtaking attack on conventional ideas of the four dimensions of space-time. Eleven dimensions were postulated—some of them "curled up" strangely. Trying to communicate intuitively the behavior of these ringed, vibrating strings, some physicists spoke of them as wriggling, wiggling, and interlacing.

I have found these metaphors greatly helpful for describing and explaining in the broadest way how experienced and experienceable worlds are put together. Though I cannot judge the mathematics involved in physicists' string theories, I can appreciate the hopes implied for unification and coherence in our existential and theoretical lives. We can dare to hope that we need not remain boxed up in the conventional four dimensions. That is to say, that we can do justice to the much-at-once that converges upon us from all conceivable "sides" every instant and (assuming no serious blockages) circulates through us amazingly. That is, in "cashing out" the consequences for experience of fundamental ideas of rhythm (or wave-length), harmony, and melody, we *may* realize Pythagoras's ancient vision of the marriage of physics, mathematics, music, ethics, and religion for our own time and place.

There is a danger that the possibilities may dazzle us into imbecility. But a greater danger, I feel, is to remain obdurately where we are: that is, in the grip of cemented dichotomies, prejudices, parochialisms, fears, and antagonisms. So I tarry a bit longer on what appear to be real possibilities in an age of unprecedented and breathtakingly rapid and dangerous change. Very recently, astrophysicists and cosmologists have inferred that much of the reality of the cosmos consists of enigmatic "dark energy"; they have inferred this from, for example, strange variations in the acceleration of the expansion of the known universe. In the summer of 2006, empirical confirmation of the existence of dark energy was claimed. Using a broad array of astronomical instruments to focus on an energy-event second in strength only to the big bang itself—that is, a collision of galaxies 3.4 light years distant in time and space—light and dark energy appear to have been pulled apart, leaving them differentiated. Einstein famously equated matter and energy, but as Richard Feynman, for one, has pointed out, even though we have equations for describing energy's behaviors within certain frameworks of inquiry, we still aren't sure what it *is*. The ancient question of Being or reality reemerges in a newly congenial context.

This has prompted certain physicist-engineer-therapists to speculate that we are bathed perpetually in potentially healing energies and vibrations that we cannot yet clearly conceive or imagine (see, for example, books by William Tiller, such as *Science and Human Transformation: Subtle Energies, Intentionality and Consciousness*, or Richard Gerber's *Vibrational Medicine: The #1 Handbook of Subtle-Energy Therapies*; one must critically inspect all this, of course, but it shouldn't be dismissed out of hand). These energies are sometimes termed "subtle," or much more problematically, "higher." Higher than what, we must ask? There is always the danger of mind/body, physical/spiritual, high-as good/low-as-bad polar oppositions that block or sidetrack, as Peirce would say, the course of inquiry into this one, mysterious, actual cosmos. Most dangerous and insidious of all is talk of "bridging the inner and the outer." What is facilely called "the inner" is just our own bodies focally communing with themselves while bobbing in the ocean of intercirculating energies consigned to the margins or fringes of awareness. As the physicist John Wheeler once put it to similarly advanced colleagues, "There's no *out there* out there." I deal further with hydra-like Cartesian dualism below.

William Tiller speculates in the following way, for example. Einstein's famous formula $e=mc^2$ should really be written over a divisor, which is the Lorenz transformation equation that reads, in English: as something approaches the speed of light, mass gets heavier and time dilates. It has been thought by most physicists that c, the speed of light, must be an absolute, since anything over that speed equals a square root of a negative number, which can only be a so-called imaginary number. For Tiller this is a prejudice. Such numbers denote actual energic realities (Tiller, *Science and Human Transformation*). Such speculations potentially open the door to radical new therapies, therapies that at least seem radical when counterpoised to the traditional, inertial background of Newtonian mechanics and the notion of the human body as a machine. The human body has five main "inlets" for sensation and perception. The new radically organismic view of the body, however, posits that it is an active porous membrane packed with intercirculating organs and a blood supply brimming with hormones and neuropeptides, one that responds resonantly as a whole to a host of impinging influences. A body, that is, responsive to the much-at-once.

Consider two examples of this: aromatherapy and osteocranial therapy. Aromatherapy exploits the fact that only some of the stimulants that reach the olfactory bulb of the brain, transposed in energy, ever affect the cerebral cortex and the possibility of conscious, reflexive, articulable recognition. Olfactory memories, while recognizable as memories, present the remembered as somehow "lived through again." The relativity and elasticity of time is directly experienced. The intensity of the original experience is reproduced. The implication is that we do not simply leave the past behind as a train leaves behind a station. One aim of such therapy is to help liberate people who may be fixated on a crushing and humiliating past event by restoring the flow of regenerative energies in, through, and out of the body (see Wilshire, *Wild Hunger: The Primal Roots of Modern Addiction*, Chapter 9).

The second example, osteocranial therapy, treats the head not just as a box with various key openings in it, but as an oh-so-alive and bony member of the whole resonating body-in-environment. Blockages here are particularly frequent and virulent, in large part because we have no direct awareness of the brain, nor of failures to resonate with the much-at-once that can occur in it. I deal with this further in the next segment, and also with my own experience as a subject in osteocranial therapy, an adjunct of Rolfing.

William James had a sharp ear for what he called the "bass-notes of life" within the various harmonies and dissonances of much-at-once sensuous experiencing. This musical metaphor hauntingly opens up key truths of experience. Bass notes are basic, are abiding bases for what is to be built on and around them. As noted earlier, John Dewey maintained in his *Logic* (1938) that foundational to all inquiry is the discernment of the felt quality of the whole situation in which inquiry is to occur. Whereto does this quality tend, to what does its vibrational reality conduce? What is this nisus, this incipient nudging or directing toward what horizon of possibilities—or toward what is tacitly taken to be impossibilities? How does this felt quality tend to turn or bend our attention toward alluring consummation on the dawning horizons of awareness? Or how does it tend to block it?

Contemporary physicists leap and fly in primal attunements, only sometimes touching down in empirical verifications. There is an analogue to this in the shuttling weavings of music. Some passages are directly evocative of primordial bodily realities, and the music builds on these, bringing the palpability to our senses. The primal excitement of rapid and frenetic beats evokes the excited beating of the heart; the soothing legato of other passages is like falling toward sleep; passages blurring-downward or swooning are very like, yes, swooning, and so on. These abuttings with directly sensed bodily realities, these direct couplings and cominglings, analogize empirical verifications in science. Other passages in music evoke the far-reaching swooping lines and targetings of human speculation and theorizing: the feeling tones of alert human bodies incident upon such activities. These analogize especially the leaps and flights in recent science, which touch down in empirical verification we know not where.[1] Each medium is a honeyed spinning and coherence: Each domain of activity resonates with and furthers the others, even if only subliminally and ineffably. We exist immersed in an oceanic, mysterious universe. We cannot fathom why it exists at all.

As we proceed and fresh horizons find us, it is only poetic justice that we be led at times by Native Americans. The New World's version of colonizing and invading European imperialism, the corporate individual

1. In speaking of his theory of relativity, Einstein wrote to a fellow mathematician Jacques Hadamard, "It occurred to me by intuition, and music was the driving force behind that intuition. My discovery was the result of musical perception." And again, "If I were not a physicist, I would probably be a musician. I often think in music. I live my daydreams in music. I see my life in terms of music" (Hadamard, *The Psychology of Invention in the Mathematical Field*, 142–43). These often-cited quotations deserve our consideration because, given all that we know about his scientific work, it makes sense that Einstein would have uttered them. Sound is less infected with treacherous unexamined presuppositions than is sight. When thought is dominated by vision and visual metaphors, it is fairly easy to think of space, for example, as a kind of huge container that might conceivably be completely empty, and to conceive of time as a kind of track that might conceivably have nothing rolling along it. These Newtonian notions of absolute space and time are pivotally rejected by Einstein, for whom space and time are real only relative to what is actually happening, immediately as it is happening for us, embedded in the much-at-once—regardless of how strange this may seem to mechanistic physics and also to common sense. One grasps fairly easily how music may have helped Einstein to understand this. For the value of any musical sound is determined by how it relates to what else is actually happening sound-wise—or has happened or is expected to happen—and to nothing else within the span of attention relative to a specific culture's "duration of a piece of music." A music empty of all sound would make no sense, whereas a space and time empty of all things happening in it or through it at least seems to make sense. Here John Cage's experimentations are revealing; when he sits down at a piano and makes no sound, this can express the very limit of *music* because he has staged a situation in which we expect him to make musical sound.

bound to the project of conquest and following the "manifest destiny" of taking over this land, could not participate in the worlds-as-experienced generated by Native American groups. Waves of expansionist-inspired, superiorly weaponed whites could only conquer and repress Native American groups. True, our best thinkers—such as Thoreau, Emerson, Peirce, James, Dewey—with antennae receptive and quivering, picked up vibrations from these indigenous groups. These particular whites knew that imperialism skated on thin ice: They knew intuitively that the destruction wreaked upon the community of peoples, animals, and lands might one day rebound upon those committing this massive violation, leaving them to live within a damaged world (see Wilshire, *Get 'Em All! Kill 'Em!: Genocide, Terrorism, Righteous Communities*). But such perceptive whites were very few, and even today they are widely ignored even by thinkers who fancy themselves informed. The expansionist ethos rolls on; technological trance and obsession rolls on with it, as does fascination with whatever is new and "news." Those able to discern what is actually happening notice startling convergences taking shape, which may lead to a summit from which a commanding new vantage point on the Whole will emerge. Or, might it be more revealing to ask, may we find ourselves in a situation in which to better *hear* what is happening?

I have already sought to retrieve and be retrieved by Black Elk. One of his cousins was the famous warrior and prophet Crazy Horse. The name does not imply that Crazy Horse was crazy, nor that his horse was. It connotes the revealing way in which his horse appeared to him. It shimmered and vibrated crazily. That is, in some sense Crazy Horse discerned what contemporary physics has discovered: that things do not exist as isolated individuals enclosed within the envelope of their surfaces, but rather they irradiate each other, participating in whole fields of energy exchanges. Similarly, in string theory, strings function as interlacing vibrating rings that transmit—sympathetically, for example—across whole vast fields. Can we say, perhaps, that we seek the tuning fork of the cosmos?

Even the possibility of a convergence of human endeavors healing the fragmentation and splintering of the contemporary world is powerfully alluring. Human attitudes and emotions of all sorts are indissociable from interlacing vibrations of bodies in fields. Perhaps we are not fated to be split between mind and body, or thought and feeling, or between individual and group, or one group against another, between human and animal. We are not fated, that is, if we can think and feel our way out of entrenched individualism on both the individual and group levels. If we can grope our way out of attendant polarizations and oppositions, which means out of attendant hierarchical habits: the prejudice of esteeming one thing superior to another by essential nature, like the prejudice that "mind" is superior to body. Mindless individualism dies hard, if it dies at all. Something as apparently innocuous as numbering things tends not to be truly innocuous since, under the Cartesian sway—the admonition to distrust our senses, discount emotions, and trust in the power of quantification as yielding true insight into the world—we are impelled to think and feel mindlessly in terms of separation, not in terms of continuousness and contiguity. We are misled in asking the question: Where does that singular thing end and another begin? Thus masked out initially and automatically are corporate unities and webbings, fields, vibrating interfusings and rhythmic intercirculatings. When these are masked out, we have already wandered into a deep obliviousness, a fragmentation of the world and ourselves.

For Black Elk, and presumably Crazy Horse, we exist within a far-flung community of beings—a real *community*, not a spurious one as that word is carelessly used today—in which the two-leggeds live in *conviviality* with the four-leggeds, the flying, hopping, striding, slithering, and swimming ones. Fragmentation isn't just occurring in "worldviews"; it happens within our bodies as discordances and disconnects that leave the interweaving circuits of energy exchanges, the emotional circuitry, in tatters and shorted. The result is emotional and existential emptiness and flatness. All along I have emphasized vibrational attunements that defy explanation in terms of traditional Western intellectualism: for example, shouting a secret to the stone. There are vibrational attunements—between stones, say, or between mountains and the sinews, nerves, and bones of our own bodies—those attunements that defy traditional conceptualization and discriminations in words. Reflection, notes James, comes too late, and catches only the crumbs that fall from the feast. The feast is our immediate, streaming caught-up-ness in the much-at-once moment by moment.

In his later work James grew wary of the very word *consciousness*, for it implies that our awareness is essentially self-reflexive, awareness of awareness, as Descartes indeed thought it was. But this is a serious mistake. Reflexiveness happens for us only sometimes and under certain conditions. To be drawn into this trap is to be severed from our nonhuman kin and the mineral world, and to invite excruciating loneliness. James coined the word *sciousness*, as Whitehead later coined *prehension*, to be distinguished from apprehension. So misleading is *consciousness*! I regard the fugal structure of the prereflective processual self as basic, but this fundamental insight can be vitiated by mindless fixating that equates awareness and reflexiveness. Or worse, that equates this with the "real self" and occludes the reality of our *bodily* being, caught up in immediacy and exhibiting tendencies and nises (plural of nisus). So insidious are our categorizing words, which enforce and reinforce the literal (alphabetic) tradition that entrenches us. Indeed, what is known as contemporary information overload—the problem of brains that "can't think" due to too much data coming in—actually stems from brains looking at, taking in, and processing the *word*. It comes from relying on seeing to give us what we need to know, when the truth is that relying on seeing *limits* what we know. Lost are the primal icons and indexes, sound-signs and symbols, the nearly vanished world of orality—all of which release us into a more open encounter with the world and its depths.

Please note, when I speak of the fugal retention in immediacy of what the retained *itself retained*, the reader will, understandably, *reflect* on his or her awareness to consider if what I say is true. But in finding this to be true, say, he or she powerfully tends to think that the fugal self is essentially reflexive. No, the fugal self holds retentions and expectations that very probably can never be perceived and brought to verbal acknowledgement by itself. Perhaps only others who observe with crafty and tenacious artistry can do this. Thus Saul Bellow, for example, in his novel *The Adventures of Augie March,* reveals an otherwise unacknowledgeable strain or vibration in the passive, feckless, apparently simple mother who was abandoned by her husband, Augie's father. "Her thoughts were always simple; but she felt abandonment, and greater pains than conscious mental ones put a dark streak to her simplicity" (9).

By way of a cautionary note, however, we live in a psychiatrized age, or what William Barrett calls an age of psychobabble, in which we find a category of pathology described as "being in a fugue state"—a way of tending to disconnect from present and actual reality. This extrapolates itself wildly beyond the categories of clinical practice. I hope it is amply clear that my use of the musical structure of fugue as a metaphor for the weaving of self through the much-at-once is the very opposite of disconnection or fragmentation within the much-at-once! The new horizons being sketched in this book are all about healing and reattunement, though this is not to say that we have an obvious, pinpointable, easily detectable pathology or disease. The very nature of the disease tends to hide itself: emotional flatness, grayness, unaliveness, boredom, sprawls out indefinitely far, a steamrollered uniformity and torpid acceptance leaves no sore thumb to be noticed. How can consciousness "expand," as some implore that it do, given that it is knotted in on itself in its very self-conception?

Contrary to what one might think, cemented atomism and self-constricted individualism do not lead to an experience of the variety of things, the sparkling suchness and just-so-ness of each thing. Just the reverse: To think that one is isolated, separated, contributes to the sense that nothing touches and moves one. It contributes to James's sheathed-in-India-rubber feeling. It's all going on "out there," and who could really care much? This standing in opposition to the world reveals a limited view of it, as compared to entering into its depths and taking in new senses through immersion.

Stopping at the surface of things is part of a new tendency, a new sort of nihilism that emerges and congeals around us in our isolation from the world and others. If formerly the nihilist believed that there is nothing really to believe in, the neonihilist doesn't gather the energy to believe even that. Comfort, convenience, the most rudimentary pleasurable sensations become by default the highest values. If one could gather the energy to scream, one would scream—but there is only deadly quiet or mindless babble. Thoreau wrote of the silent desperation into which we moderns tend to fall.

The first need is to be awakened. String theorists have been awakened by having the contradictions of conventional science thrust, so to speak, in their faces. Great artists have always tried to awaken themselves and others. Novel strokes have animated their brushes, chisels, pens, fingertips on instruments, their whole, animating, moving bodies. The wakeup call is a shocking, vibrating, tympanic thing. It may even come with what Bugbee calls true silence—when distractions lose their grip for a moment and the Whole flows into us, enlivening us. Miracle of miracles, we are found as beings who were once fetuses floating in amniotic fluid. We experience a mysterious birth, or rebirth. Whatever truly finds us and claims us sets us a-vibrating. Once animated, we may come alive to hang-ups and fixations and disconnects that had previously been smothered in cotton padding. We may then profit from vibrations of endless sorts that may reattune and reinvigorate us—new, beneficent trances.

More and more palpably the trance of the American Dream is broken into by a generalized restlessness—at least for those who still feel anything. The spell of the commercial, secular, technological trance is unsettled and disrupted for quite a few. Just finding a true alternative to the sprawling, routine, gray state—some enlivening variety, some depth in being alive—is imperative. Once again, to quote Felicitas Goodman, we cannot long tolerate ecstasy deprivation. Thinking that we can easily leads to all kinds of desperate addictions, not only to drugs but to obsessive overwork (workaholism) and the endless amassing of wealth. Anything but meaninglessness and emptiness, death in life! If a hidden spark or burning ember of life bursts into flame, we may find ourselves echoing Crazy Horse rallying his men and women to rub out Custer: "It's a good day to fight, it's a good day to die!" A tedious lament may erupt into that! That *reality!*

In a time like this, we should not be surprised to find appearing a book like Gerber's *Vibrational Medicine.* Some of his examples are crude, yet true enough. Two tuning forks pitched to the same frequency: If one is struck into sounding, the other picks up and sounds with that frequency. In forks only close to the same pitch, this does not occur. The application to therapy is obvious. If one resonates only to negativity, if one has habitually been found only by what is life-denying, then therapy has to identify the vibrations that repitch one into affirmation. This approach opens out onto Goodman's work on ecstatic-reverential trance postures, which she has discovered in many different places on earth (Goodman, *Where the Spirits Ride the Wind: Trance Journeys and Other Ecstatic Experiences*). The assumption of these trance postures by adepts is always accompanied by the rhythmical beating of drums or shaking of rattles: a kind of hypnosis, as we might say, that can free one to new ways of being—good trances in this case.

It is astonishing to witness the tidal strength of the need and urge for repitching or reattuning now abroad in the world. To my knowledge, none is more extreme than that espoused and broadcast by Masuru Emoto in *The True Power of Water: Healing and Discovering Ourselves*. In a short time, he has become a world-girdling phenomenon as lecturer and author. Should he have this influence? Succinctly summarized, he has developed a method for photographing ice crystals as they appear in frozen water. Astonishingly, if he is to be believed, they appear to be profoundly influenced not only by chemically analyzable pollutants but also by human attitudes toward them.

Now, since we have done our best in this book to overwhelm traditional dualistic and atomistic splits and schisms—that is, ones that isolate "minds" vis-à-vis bodies—we should not just dismiss this possibility out of hand. As the reality of Crazy Horse's horse was not bottled up and contained within the envelope of its surfaces, but radiated and shimmered outward, why shouldn't human attitudes be construed as radiating from human bodily beings into what is irradiated? And since some attitudes are loving and respectful while others are neglectful or contemptuous, why shouldn't we suspect that the former are affirming of crystals and conduce to their being well formed and beautiful, whereas the latter might distort and deform them? Emoto's photographs provide what he takes to be proof of this. He builds a kind of theoretical structure within which attitudes are conceived to involve the subatomic level of human bodily selves and to act on the subatomic level of water. If true, we have taken a giant step toward discovering a new community for our world, toward reviving a new Pythagorean vision of the unity of science and ethics, of mind and matter, of science and art. The reader of Emoto's book will enjoy at its close his account of the fundamental causal properties of different pieces of music. In short, if true, we are on the verge of discovering a true and responsible worldwide religion that commands our passion and commitment.

But is it true? Might it be a sham and a hoax, or more likely, perhaps, a desperate wish-fulfillment fantasy for a world perilously close to extinction? Scientists, and not just conventional ones, will want to ask questions. Why not conduct double-blind experiments to test these claims? (Would Emoto think that the impersonality of these would negatively influence the formation of crystals under observation? To my knowledge, he does not say.) Is the formation of crystals susceptible only to *human* influences? How about the influence of a deer sipping at a pool? Could a container of frozen water exhibit a wide variety of crystals, among which one could "cherry pick" evidence on the basis of one's interest in the theory? Questions need to be pressed. But the issues are so crucial that we should not commit the intellectually unforgivable sin of blocking or impeding the road of inquiry, as Charles Peirce would again put it.

So far I have related science and music mainly in schematic and general ways, barely sketching a few concrete therapies, but the concrete interrelations of science and music are practically endless. For a few decades now there have been scientific studies of the nervous system, particularly the brain, when the organism is involved in experiencing music. These should be encouraged. Yet, as already intimated, there is a danger of premature concentration on the brain itself, which is to mask out the whole changing, vibrating, porous body in its changing, vibrating, encompassing environment. That is, even if the Cartesian notion of the isolated private consciousness is longer explicitly affirmed, the privileged locus it formerly occupied has been filled by the stopgap of the isolated, encapsulated brain—a perverse and ironic equivalence. The ghost of the strange reified entity the *mind* now incarnates itself as the *brain*. Amazing how deeply rooted are old-fashioned notions of mechanism, self-enclosing atoms and atomism, and mind/body polar oppositions or dualisms (see again my note on Peirce and the attempt to locate the mind, Segment 5, note 3).

We can keep expanding our metaphor of the fugue-like self in its vibrational reality. Our lives hang together over time because of organized sequences of activity that are repeatable. They may be retained or recollected in focal awareness, or they may be repeated through "muscle memory"—the repeatable resonances of the whole organism. We might call these repeated organized sequences basic units of meaning—or even better, body-meaning. Our bodies move in primal ways, and the various timings and degrees of urgency in our actions and soundings form paradigmatic repeatable *rhythms*. When the pitch of our actions—including our speech and all the sounds we make—is modulated in distinctively organized and repeatable ways, we get paradigmatic *melodies*.

For example, it is not just verbally formulated questions that end on a higher pitch, but our whole inquiring bodies are up, looking around, hoping for resolution and answers. Nor is it arbitrary that when on urgent alert—in emergency situations—our bodily state involves a certain breathlessness and constriction of the body, including of course the voice box. The sounds we make in these situations are typically high pitched—screams, shrieks, or whistles of expiring breath.

As logocentric beings we tend to hypostatize or "nounify" our capacities, as if they were things or possessions—"mind," "speech," and so on—but underlying all these artifacts of verbalizable and writable language, and nearly hidden by them, are the primal bodily processes that repeat, that make and remake themselves. In an appropriately broad sense we can call this primal music-making—indeed, as something *made*. Since we are agents, selves, we also *make* some of it. That is, endemic to our sense of ourselves enduring through time is our sense of ourselves as initiators of meaningful patterns of activity. In some individuals, such as Jefferson and Peirce, the need to initiate distinctive—even revolutionary—patterns of activity is so overwhelming that may leave them exhausted, or racked with incapacitating headaches. Relative to conventional standards of meaningful conduct, sclerotic as they are, these persons are unstable. The price of genius is extremely high.

Still, these warnings about isolating the brain should not stop scientific investigators from studying it as an essential stage in ongoing organism–environment circulations and exchanges of energy. For many years it has been known that different areas of the brain provide necessary conditions for specific sensuous capacities: The occipital area in the back of the brain, for example, is necessary for vision, the temporal at the sides of the brain are necessary for hearing. Knowledge of such necessary conditions sometimes derives from studying brain-injured patients, as when, for instance, a soldier's shot-away occipital lobe results in blindness. But there is a grave danger in mistaking necessary conditions for sufficient ones. Without necessary conditions a sensuous capacity cannot be realized, but such conditions being present is not sufficient for the capacity to be realized. Sufficiency requires a whole functioning body in a whole functioning environment to which the organism can adapt. As John Dewey put it, the basic unit cannot be brain alone, but brain-in-body-in-environment: All functions must flow in concert with the others.

The brain has proved to be much more malleable than it was imagined to be not so long ago. As a crucial stage in a whole interactive circuit, the brain has taken the forms that it has needed to take for the whole organism to survive. It receives impact from every side, every moment, and repeated patterns of impact and habitual patterns of satisfaction of need are either accommodated and retained by the species' brain over the generations or the organism dies. The environment is an evolving matrix into which the brain must fit.

Brain science has become a vast and rapidly expanding field of inquiry, aided in large part by sophisticated new monitors and scans of the brain (which are nonetheless still very crude, I'm afraid). Areas of the brain laid down very probably in prehuman creatures are still carried with us today, and mapping interactive patterns is an awesome challenge that researchers are beginning to chip away at. See, for example, work by Joseph LeDoux on the primitive brain organ, the amygdala, which picks up threats in the surround through fear responses many thousandths of a second before they can be acknowledged—if they ever are—in the focus of consciousness (*Synaptic Self: How Our Brains Become Who We Are*). That is, there is much beyond what we can *say* goes on in our functioning bodies that nevertheless has primal and decisive meaning for our life in the world.

That all human cultures have music suggests strongly that, in its various forms, music is necessary for survival and for vital life. If this is so, it must be because music coordinates matters that must be coordinated, and this can be done in no other way. I mean music not reduced in our understanding to merely neural-electrical discharges in the temporal lobes of the brain, but music as the whole vibratory, moving, patterning body: what we call *dance*—that which develops germinally from the tapping of feet or the drumming of fingertips, and so on. That there is incredibly much to coordinate also suggests that mal-coordination is an ever-present possibility and a very frequent actuality. A florid form of self-deception—disastrous in some circumstances—is to allow an activity to go on because one's attention has been deflected to some remote topic or activity (compare Jean-Paul Sartre's example, in *Being and Nothingness,* of a woman allowing herself to be seduced in this fashion). The destructive effects of distraction and fragmentation on the life of the corporate body seem far greater than we realize.

Emerson's insight, quoted earlier, could not be more germane: In poetry it is precisely the breathing of the body, in whatever mobilization and rhythm, that gives birth to the words, so that deep coordination is achieved. Again I quote:

> We are lovers of rhyme and return, period and musical reflection. . . . Metre begins with pulse-beat, and the length of lines in songs and poems is determined by the inhalation and exhalation of the lungs. If you hum or whistle the rhythm of the common English metres . . . you can easily believe these metres to be organic, derived from the human pulse. . . . I think you will . . . be at once set on searching for the words that can rightly fill these vacant beats. ("Poetry and Imagination," 8:24–25)

True, this coordination may be achieved only while the poetry is being written or heard, but still, great values are garnered. First, there is the relief of dislocation healed, if only temporarily; we are retuned and reattuned as whole organisms. Second, matters dislocated or repressed may be evoked in the poetic art—given its "aesthetic distance"—that we could not bear to acknowledge in raw life. Although artistic experience might all too easily become an evasive substitute for such deep acknowledgement and lasting behavioral change, it may just as easily supply the momentary insight and equilibration that leads to that acknowledgement. It all depends how seriously one is stanced to dig into the truth of one's life when opportunity presents itself. Here aesthetics verges uncertainly on ethics and character. We remember John Dewey's astonishing remark in *Art as Experience* that "art is more moral than moralities" (348).

The brain is much more plastic, porous, susceptible than the standard ideology cemented by mind/body dualism, atomism, and mechanism inclines us to think. As I've said, the brain is just one complex stage in the circuits of energy exchanges running throughout whole-organism-in-whole-environment. Research on the two hemispheres of the brain, for example, has led some to conclude that the right hemisphere in right-handed people is much more intuitive and emotional than is the left. Given the "crossover" in the nervous system regarding right and left sides, emotionally loaded music fed into the left ear—hence into the right-brain hemisphere—of people who are not musically trained is more apt to be remembered than if it is fed into the right ear (see John Sloboda, *The Musical Mind: The Cognitive Psychology of Music*, 264). But for musicians, who grasp the structure of the music intellectually, when it is fed into their left versus right ears, this does not hold, so intimately are their two brain hemispheres adjusted to the whole situation, due to the personal-historical development of the organism in question. (Here it's worth noting, with the oddness and precarious balance of genius, Charles Peirce considered himself disadvantaged because he was left-handed.)

How widely involved is the brain! A highly suggestive though not conclusive indication of this is found in the embryology of the human nervous system. At a certain stage of the development of the fetus, that which becomes the skin of the organism differentiates itself as the brain. There is some reason to assert, then, that the skin is the surface of the brain (*Creation Spirituality*, May/June, 1991). This reminds us of all that rains in on the brain. Included are neuropeptides generated in various parts of the body, fluctuating in league with changing circumstances and carried by the bloodstream supplying the brain (see writings of Candace Pert, e.g., *The Molecules of Emotion: Why You Feel the Way You Feel*).

As the brain functions in the whole body living in the whole environment, so does the heart. More influences, more stimuli, rain in on the functioning organism from any natural environment than could ever be described, let alone predicted. Ingredient in vital life is spontaneity and chance, and the heart is an essential node in this fluxing field of energy exchanges—of thoughts, feelings, emotional transports, trances. Great art brings bubbling surprises that not only delight, but are vital nourishment for the heart in supplying it with a rich brew of emotions and feelings.

Because the heart is directly felt in the flux of alerted emotional life, we may think that it is *the* seat of the emotions. As it bangs away in the chest cavity and ribs, its role is unmistakable, whereas by contrast the brain cannot be directly experienced, and we are apt to think of it as locked away in the strongbox of the skull, "making calculations" perhaps. But both organs resonate with the power of music's rhythms, emotional expressions, and melodies.

The cardiologist Ari Goldberger has translated the different features of electrocardiograms into sequences of sounds and pitches (see David Suzuki, *The Sacred Balance*, episode 1). He then contrasts the music of healthy hearts with that made by those damaged by heart failure. The music of healthy hearts is rich, complex, never totally predictable; that of damaged hearts is monothematic, mechanical, flat and boring. With the healthy heart, it's as if one were listening to different streams intertwining in confluence: one hears chance concordances, even some passing discords, and surprising blips, sparkles, isomorphisms and augmentations that stand out a bit as they pass. It's creatively fugal (note, in comparison, the quintuple inverted counterpoint of the last movement of Mozart's last symphony, the *Jupiter*, particularly the trumpet part). The damaged heart plugs away, the essentials of bare survival met, but with none of the play, joy, creativity, and spontaneity of vital life. So the inner life of the body may be understood as in musical interplay with the outer world.

Transdisciplinary research shouldn't be especially remarkable, but given the segmenting and cementing effects of hyper-specialized inquiry, it is—and always present are the deleterious effects of mind/matter dualisms. Various polar oppositions and dualisms that rule thought today, coupled with the hyperspecialization and professionalization of academic research, have badly obscured the cohesiveness and creative continuity of our lives. Shakespeare very frequently uses iambic meters in his poetic rendering of dramatic human life. The iambic meter is one subdued beat followed by an accented one. Many of his lines are five such meters in succession, iambic pentameter. Though it should not surprise us, it often does, that iambic meter directly conveys the beating of the heart, its systole and diastole: the da-DA, da-DA, da-DA. When the warrior Macbeth tries to face down his wife's charge that he is a coward, the abruptness of the iambics directly renders his defiance, and his terrible fear that he has been cornered in a dastardly adventure:

> *I dare do all that may become a man;*
> *Who dares do more is none.*
> (*Macbeth*, act 1, sc. 7)

We would be greatly remiss not to mention scientific work on brain waves and the relevance of music to these studies (see the work of the adventurous physician Andrew Weil along with Kimba Arem, *Self-Healing with Sound and Music*). Four common brainwave frequencies have been identified through the use of electroencephalograms: alpha, beta, delta, theta. The brain generates all these frequencies simultaneously, but the ratio between the frequencies varies from moment to moment. Brain studies of high-performance people in many fields suggest that certain brainwave patterns and ratios of the four types are associated with "an awakened mind or optimum state." The researchers endeavor to use sound creatively to produce this optimal mix of brainwaves through the process of entrainment. This is the phenomenon wherein various bodily processes—heart rate, brainwaves, respiration—synchronize with the frequencies of what we hear. Attesting, once again, that inner body and outer world are interwoven musically.

In an especially valuable section of the CDs, Kimba Arem connects her studies of indigenous healing traditions with these brainwave studies. She speaks of expanded states of consciousness that promote healing. One can only be heartened by these expanded horizons of research. Still, one must be constantly vigilant lest unexamined European, particularly Cartesian, assumptions leak into the analyses and vitiate the conclusions; the very idea of "states of consciousness" can do this. It can artificially isolate "the experiencing subject," trapping it in a tunnel vision, masking off the actual brain-in-body-in-environment, the intercirculating total unit of reality. Moreover, this unit must be stretched out through time and place if the healing synchrony is not to be merely momentary. We are habitual beings whose health requires continuity through time and entrainment through reliable rituals.

What is more, the synchrony must be widened to include communion with beings beyond our own species. Indigenous people may well remind us of this. In her remarkable novel *Ceremony*, Leslie Marmon Silko writes of returning war veteran Tayo, the child of a Native American and an Anglo. His life had been shattered. Two events begin to reconnect him. A healer places him squatting on a floor as all around him a sand painting of the cosmos as the Native American people understand it is gradually composed. Tayo sees himself "found" at his own place and time in the Whole (since we are writing of the sacred all-togetherness of things, we should capitalize this). Thus Tayo's disabling fear is addressed with some effect. In the second connecting event, far out in the arid mountains with only a moon's light to see by and wind in his face, Tayo happens upon a mountain lion suddenly in a clearing before him. Tayo gets to his knees, looks into the animal's eyes, orbs that catch twin reflections of the moon, and whispers, "Mountain lion, mountain lion, becoming what you are with each breath, your substance changing with the earth and sky." The narrative goes on, "The mountain lion blinked his eyes; there was no fear." Then like liquid deflected, the lion turns and goes its way silently, disappearing into the trees. Tayo, who had collapsed in exhaustion and pain before the lion's approach, afterward feels revitalized as if he has returned to himself from being lost.

What concord sounds here? What supplanting of disabling fear? Leslie Silko is wrenching open dominant white-American culture of the twentieth century. In placing the half-breed, war-shattered Tayo within a context of Native American healing practices, she opens the dominant culture to new possibilities, but not painlessly. For the dominant culture must question the assumptions that it has taken completely for granted: that we are the ministers of progress on our planet, that the global conflict that North American or Euro-American culture engenders is somehow really for the best. Greatly creative people outstrip the standards for evaluating human performance that operate at any given time within a culture. They wrench open the culture, at some cost to those who do it (as we have seen in the genius of Jefferson and Peirce). Those who perform well within the culture as it stands may very well exhibit harmony among their various brain wave patterns, but it is unlikely, I think, that creative geniuses will show this. Studies are called for; perhaps we should expect strong dissonances in these extraordinarily creative few!

In any case, it should be clear that examination of brainwave patterns alone cannot supply the criteria for evaluating the work of extraordinary "high-performance" people; we must see the whole picture, see "performance" in the broadest scope. The criteria of excellence must be those kinds of work that further the real enlightenment and actual welfare of humanity and fellow species. The atomistic notion of inspecting and exhibiting "the brain" in isolation cannot pan out, nor can the Cartesian notion of inspecting and reporting "the mind" alone. As the exploratory stage artist Peter Brook writes:

> All through human history, every society ends up by getting it wrong. In the beginning there is always a bold rush of energy. This creates new, fresh structures, but they soon turn into institutions, which from then on slowly become fossils. This process unfortunately is human. ("About *Tierno Bokar*")

Nietzsche was disturbed by the displacements of human beings from the matrix of the encompassing environment that formed us for hundreds of thousands of years. He was disturbed to the point of thinking that the brain must be chemically or surgically altered. Nor was he daunted by the ridicule that had come to surround nineteenth-century attempts to alter the brain through encasing it, for example, in magnets. Indeed, interventions in the brain are legion. The more things change, apparently quixotically, the more they remain the same. Thus, more recently we hear of repetitive transcranial magnetic stimulation (rTMS), the point of which is to heal dislocations within the brain. It has become clear that neurons in different parts of the brain can act in concert. Particularly notable are the circuits that link the various areas of the cortex that enable us to reason and plan with the more deeply embedded zones of the brain, such as the limbic system where emotions are processed. One theory claims that depression results from an imbalance in the activity within those regions. Applying periodic bursts of electrical current at the cortex may reset the network in a process that resembles rebooting a computer. Some depressed patients have been helped by this technique.

I think that an imbalance in the brain is most often the resultant microcosm of an imbalance in the whole brain-in-body-in-environment circulatory unit, the macrocosm. This intricately functioning much larger unit is the fruit of countless millennia of the formation of the species through adaptation to Nature's environments by hunting-gathering-scavenging. Very many today are so greatly dislocated from these home environments that intervening directly in the brain may be the only recourse, but if that is the case, we should at least be aware of our desperate straits, and aware that cures achieved thereby may well be only temporary, in need of continuing readjustment. This, of course, is not to dismiss these therapeutic methods, nor to minimize the urgent needs addressed.

One of the major surprises of contemporary physics occurred in the 1920s with disclosures of the strange behavior of microscopic particles within the atom. Their behaviors could not be determined with mechanical certainty (see Niels Bohr, Werner Heisenberg, and so-called quantum mechanics). Chance and randomness figured importantly: The best that could be predicted about these microscopic particles were probabilities of paths and distributions. But it was thought for a while that a gulf lay between these odd, microscopic behaviors within the atom and the gross, macroscopic level of reality in which we live our everyday lives. This idea has been radically altered—even prescinding from new string theories for the moment. Quite recently the physicist Roger Penrose, for example, has speculated in *The Emperor's New Mind: Concerning Computers, Minds and the Laws of Physics* and *Shadows of the Mind: A Search for the Missing Science of Consciousness* that the microtubules of the brain's neurons may be sufficiently numerous and tiny to allow quantum phenomena to occur within our own bodies. What role does chance and randomness play in our own lives, most particularly in the lives of the most creative of us? Note that Peirce believed that chance and randomness are real, that their appearance is not always due merely to ignorance of causes.

It is possible, of course, to be too unstable. But it is also possible to be too stable for great creativity. As in the cases of the genius of Peirce and Jefferson, is there an optimal degree of instability—so that one stays open to productive randomness, open to how one happens to be found (in the sense of *Befindlichkeit*)? Must one be unstable enough for true creativity? The presumed gulf between micro and macro realities has been bridged in still other ways, and indeed these studies are more advanced than are Penrose's speculations concerning the need for a new quantum physics of the nervous system. Statistical studies on the strictly atomic level, for example, have inspired such studies on smallish *macroscopic* things in large groups of such things. These include studies of the behavior of ants in anthills, of ant colonies, and of bees in beehives. These studies in turn have led me to speculate that creativity in the arts and sciences may be better understood if we *radically* develop Dewey's idea that the basic unit of reality here is brain-in-body-in-environment. Is there a dynamic, creative critical mass in such a radically dilated *unit* in which chance or randomness—in just the right degree or balance—plays a decisive role?

Consider that in an ant colony, as population densities and corresponding activity levels increase, critical thresholds in the reality of the colony are crossed. These thresholds are as dramatic and abrupt as is the thirty-two-degree Fahrenheit threshold for the behavior of water: Crossing this threshold on the rise means, of course, the passage from a solid to a liquid state. When the population and activity levels of ants in the colony increase beyond a certain critical point, the whole colony changes. Ants that are not touched by other ants with a certain frequency become moribund and idle. But when, for any reason, the frequency of touching rises above the threshold, a whole new and vital rhythm of activity takes over rapidly within the colony. It produces a rhythmical humming and a buzzing, even if inaudible to our unaided ears.

A beehive presents a similar phenomenon, and one eminently audible to us. Thus in *War and Peace,* Tolstoy has a character place his ear near the hive so he can diagnose its state of health. A flat or static level of sound or only sporadic sound—little sound at all—means a sick hive, probably a queenless one.

> There is no longer the measured, quiet sound of throbbing activity . . . but diverse discordant sounds of disorder. In and out of the hive long black robber bees smeared with honey fly timidly and shiftily. They do not sting but crawl away from danger. Formerly only bees laden with honey flew into the hive, and they flew out empty; now they fly out laden. (*War and Peace,* Part III, Chapter 20, 210)

What does this have to do with human creativity? A lot, I speculate. I think that in the case of greatly creative people, the brain-in-body-in-environment functions on analogy with colonies of ants and hives of bees. For all human organisms, waves of stimuli and multifarious surrounding influences rain in on us from all directions every moment. They interact with resonances and residues already there, already carried by the organism. Some human beings go insane because, for whatever reason, they cannot tolerate the constant threat of uncertainty, disruption, violation. But most human organisms armor themselves against this by unwittingly absorbing the defensive and excluding habits of their social and cultural group. As William James put it, the continuity of the corporate body requires this, for "habit is the flywheel of society." Or, if we listen to Martin Buber:

> Each of us in encased in an armor whose task is to ward off signs. Signs happen to us without respite, living means being addressed, we would need only to present ourselves and to perceive. But the risk is too dangerous for us, the soundless thunderings seem to threaten us with annihilation, and from generation to generation we perfect the defence apparatus. (*Between Man and Man*, 10)

Now what of that very small percentage of greatly creative people? I think they possess just the right degree of instability to allow into themselves the degree of randomness or chance necessary for great creativity. That is, the environment as the much-at-once has various impacts upon us every moment that are never completely predictably. It—"the blooming, buzzing, confusion"—is analogous with the colony or hive in energetic states of activity. But, extending the analogy, when a threshold is passed, a totalizing rhythm, a throbbing humming, takes over and possesses the whole colony. For greatly creative *human* organisms it is a totalizing rhythm or humming that is *new* to the group. Occurring is a breakthrough to a new pitch of rhythm that—suddenly in a rush—washes out old cloggings, dammings, armorings, cliches, old habits. Opened up is a whole new vista of the world qua experienceable; fresh winds blow, new experiences and possibilities awaken for us. It may take a considerable time before the geniuses are recognized for their efforts, and in the meantime suffering on all sides occurs.

Greatly creative people tolerate—indeed, they ecstatically welcome—the unprethinkable. They are held tightly by no "body of knowledge." For such a body of knowledge, integral to the flywheel of society, is what has already been categorized, classified, catalogued, and found useful by the corporate body, the group. It certainly is useful, and creative people themselves most of the time rest solidly on it. But they are not held tightly by it. Great creativity is a greased, lightning-fast sliding into a startlingly new register (recall my earlier references in Segment 3 to great performances of the final movement of Beethoven's last piano sonata). Certainly, they do not create "just to be new"; the terrible snare of pursuit of novelty per se short-circuits the moving, self-collecting funding of the past in the present, that out of which all true creativity coils with its sharp intensity. True creativity springs out of how we have always already been found by the world—as captured, again, in the term *Befindlichkeit.*

Jazz at its best exhibits vividly the essential structure and dynamics of true creativity. This improvisatory making of music accepts as given the reality of traditional tonal chords, and the harmonies integral to chords, but it incites departures from anything like rigid chordal progressions of notes, and also from any strict adherence to traditional intervals of tones, such as fifths or thirds, whether major or minor. As exemplified, say, in the expert jazz pianism of Jill McManus, the piano may fly over the other instruments, picking up only occasionally a note that touches on a harmony with something below it. The musician's whole body must be attuned to what is happening instantaneously all around it, long before any calculations can be made within the focus of reflexive consciousness (Jill McManus, *Spring Is Here*).

Only occasionally will an entire melody appear, and only occasionally in the harmonies with which it first presented itself—whether in the written music itself or in the popular media. Listeners untutored in what to expect from jazz may be at a loss to see the point of it all and may ask despairingly, "But where is the melody?" It is usually there, but listeners must stretch the scope of their attention far beyond what they previously took to be its limits. New habits of attention are required, and the process of acquiring them may involve loss of comfort and convenience, may entail displeasure and frustration. The ecstasy of creation is often acquired only with the pain of stretching and reaching into the extra-ordinary.

Creativity has been essential to human survival, and a people's music is a touchstone of its creativity. Here, in this essential cultural activity, whole bodies in concert with one another exercise their sustaining freedoms, styles, skills. As mentioned in the preceding segment, the genius of African drumming and dancing found a path for itself in Central and South America when it was blocked by slaveholders in the United States. The samba animated and excited the carnival season in Argentina, for example, and probably stems from a syncretism of indigenous and African appetites and skills.

Such influences were taken up by great jazz musicians such as Dizzy Gillespie, Charlie Parker, and Stan Getz in the United States in the not-so-distant past (see Donald Maggin, *Stan Getz: A Life in Jazz*). Something was going on in jazz culture that eluded the literate, wordy, European intellect with its cemented emphasis on reflexive consciousness. Without simply dispensing with bars (say in three-quarter time), Dizzy Gillespie played fast and loose within them. He improvised a new way of finding himself found. As Jill McManus pointed out to me, one learns to use the bars as expert slalom skiers use the posts around which they must turn. Merely mechanical responses will not do, for the fluent and creative turn is a function of more factors inherent in time and place and body-selves than the reflecting or calculating consciousness can account for or produce. We deal with the humming, buzzing, jumping much-at-once.

The power of jazz to convey the much-at-once was forcibly evident to me in the drumming of Dan Brubeck. Clearly, many more impulses converged upon and within him than could ever be enumerated, calculated, or deliberately arranged. But in a stretch of consummate moments of playing, his upper body and head swayed back and forth in what came across as a trance that blessed us. The sound of his drummings in their spontaneity organized themselves into a rapturous whole: moments of grace for us. When, similarly, aboriginals in Australia play their didgeridoos, they conform to no bar structure. Their traditional forms of life, dictated by their Dreaming, are changed—violated—only at their extreme peril. Still, each indigenous group must find itself afresh then and there in whatever Dreaming it belongs to.

SEGMENT EIGHT

THE MIND OF MUSIC

As detailed in Part I, and augmented in this second part, the fugue in music conveys with great concision the dynamic self-compounding structure of the self. A "fuguing tune," as the American composer Henry Cowell put it, sounds, then as it recedes slightly into the momentary past, still present in experiencing, sounds a second time, and so on. This grabs our attention and secures our involvement because it speaks immediately to our experiencing. Inevitably, this ongoing weaving and repeating retention reaches into the future as well: We have expectations of more to come. Arthur Schopenhauer wrote that listeners want to hear a theme again because they don't understand what it means. The word for understanding in German is *Verstand*, which couples with its contrasting term *Vernunft*, or reason. What understanding cannot grasp and is puzzled by, reason can grasp. Schopenhauer limited understanding to the focal and wordy consciousness, which *represents* the world to whatever extent it can. Reason, on the other hand, *presents* the world directly and immediately and makes evident the will (*Wille*), the life force itself: that is, our momentum as organisms through the many moments of time. (This trenchant distinction was nicely appropriated by Emerson.) Reason deals with *intensity* and is particularly interesting for us in this book.

When Schopenhauer claims that we want to hear a theme again because we don't *understand* it, he seems to mean that our understanding is baffled and obsessively wants another crack at trying to understand it. But on a deeper level, I think, we want to hear the theme again because *reason,* presenting the theme, conveys the will (*Wille*), the life force, and this is relentlessly and necessarily repetitive. Music is the voicing or sounding of *reason*, which has its own logic; reason is at the heart of what Nietzsche calls the "mind of music." Reason demands that the theme be heard again and again because it delights in it! Through the theme, the self repeatedly and intensely comes home to itself. I think that Thomas Mann was close to this notion when he wrote that music *quickens* the experiencing of time.

The fugue is a concentrated instance or species of a larger musical structure that is also an essential structure of the human self. In fugue, we hear time and again the same theme repeated; this instances a larger structure that can be described as *simul in multis*, the same in and through the many. The *multis* can take a multitude of forms. It needn't always entail many repetitions or iterations of the same theme or sequence of notes, played so that they sound together within one stretch of present awareness. It may be the same theme played much later in a piece that nevertheless fetches up a remembering or rehearing of its earlier sounding, retrieving this earlier incarnation. It may be played with one or several instruments not used earlier, or in a plangent chord played by the full orchestra, or now in human voices, now in sounds suggesting nonhuman voices. It may be the same theme sounded, say, in pizzicato strokes. Each sort of sounding resonates with its distinctive bodily-emotional correlate in the evolving self. In his dreaming or daydreaming, for example, Robert Schumann obsessively heard "trumpets in C"; thus entranced, he composed his Second Symphony around this experience (Symphony no. 2 in C Major, op. 61), for which the trumpets are the unifying force and abiding, liberating trance.

In serious art this repetition is never merely mechanical, but always entails organic and consummatory growth. *Simul in multis*, the same in and through many, implies an evolving unification through an indefinite number and sort of individual instances or events that amount to fruition, some kind of realization—the "realizing sense of things," as Dewey put it. There will be an organic experience of spontaneity that nevertheless sounds inevitable, and this occurs on the level of *reason*, as Schopenhauer and Emerson insist, not just the level of the understanding. It needn't be articulable in words, for it is occurring on the prereflective and preanalytic level of experiencing, the primal level of ecstatic involvement in the immediately presented and viscerally engaging world. It is not at the everyday level of business affairs, of getting and spending, detachedly classifying, or tallying instances of concepts. It is our distinctive and necessary way of disclosing our kinship with the other animals and birds, the elaborate ways that they do not seem to have to master. It is our way of disclosing the life force, which otherwise simply engulfs us, too often numbingly. It is our way of breaking loose from ossified words and concepts, finding ourselves at home in otherness.

Music and the related arts do not simply "disclose the facts" as history or the conventional sciences would hope to do. For the formulation of these truths about the world inevitably entails detachment from the immediacies of total emotional and existential involvements. Indeed, as Emerson put it, this level of packageable truth and understanding must be *melted* ecstatically in the art; it must be so if the deeper structuring and self-structuring of the self in its immediate moment to moment life is to be disclosed through the minding and reasoning unique to music and its cousin arts. This is the subconscious or preconscious minding and pulsing body itself—never fully predictable.

Perhaps the best example of this gulf dividing artistic process and reasoning from inevitably wordy, prosaic, and literal understanding is that supplied by contrapuntal inversion of themes. The inverted theme mirrors the original. That is, if the original ascends in pitch one increment, the inverted one descends that one increment, and so on. Both original and inverted typically round out on the same note, though perhaps not simultaneously. Typically only persons technically trained in music can perceive and articulate when inversion is occurring. But on the level of *reasoning*, on the level of the artistically rendered life force for human bodily beings, this inversion is registered and has its effect on the attentive, even if verbally inarticulate listener—or listener-dancer-poet.

In the Final Benediction of this book I discuss the time-honored role of ritual in achieving that continuity of life that carries us through inevitable shocks and disruptions. Also pointed up are various phony and counterfeit continuities—addictions, compulsions, diabolisms—that either mimic vital, healthful continuities or that defiantly block and destroy them. Much emphasized is the role of the arts, particularly music and dance, in thematizing genuine and counterfeit continuities, as well as diabolical defiances. Indeed, it is the magic of art that it can create continuity through its very rendering of the diabolical.

We can speak of the dynamic self-structuring of the self as long as we remember securely that this self-structuring occurs within a matrix of *being-found*. Whether we can speak of it or not, it is self-structuring that goes on continuously in and through one changing environment after another. A weakness or disconnect here means a weakness or perversion of the self. Here we must add immediately that we are, in our blood and bones, social and cultural creatures. From our earliest days, we are conditioned by those others looming above and around us to share experience in patterned ways; to agree about matters in ways embedded in unquestioned norms and practices of the immediate family or intimate group—and by larger groups that to various extents subsume the smaller (see Amos Tversky and Daniel Kahneman, "Judgment Under Uncertainty: Heuristics and Biases"). Groups have a corporate identity, and this must be maintained over time by a process analogous to that by which individual persons maintain their identity through time. Social codes, themes, theories, beliefs, norms, perceptual stances, countless forms of body language are repeated, recapitulated, gradually altered over time. But the group always exhibits some basal continuity through time and some anticipation of what is to come.

We are today experiencing profound cultural fragmentation, deep disintegration in the continuity and identity of traditional groups. One hope, however slim, is that the continuity of science can help to knit together the peoples of the earth in mutual understanding and shared faith and trust. But the great strengths of science entail a sobering weakness: the inevitable degree of detachment from minute-to-minute streaming life that science at some points necessitates. A less obvious aspect of this detachment is that science, as Dewey observed, is the art of making precise predictions. This virtue exacts a price, which is that immediate experiencing in all its flowing qualitative richness cannot be precisely predicted or even described—and predictions of probability miss the point, for we always remain individual beings at unique intersections of space-time. As a consequence, immediate experiencing tends to be masked out. There is no substitute for the direct experiencing of qualitative richness and reality, moment to moment, here and now, which is never more evident than in listening to music. Einstein was well aware of this, as his biographer Ronald W. Clark suggests:

> Albert Einstein was asked one day by a friend "Do you believe that absolutely everything can be expressed scientifically?" "Yes, it would be possible," he replied, "but it would make no sense. It would be description without meaning—as if you described a Beethoven symphony as a variation in wave pressure." (Clark, *Einstein: The Life and Times,* quoted in David Suzuki, *The Sacred Balance: Rediscovering Our Place in Nature*, 33)

The United States is currently suffering a collective identity crisis, and this affects all, or nearly all, of its citizens. Since our very being requires participation in the ongoing life of groups, corporate individuals, this crisis negatively affects the ability of individual citizens to knit-up their lives as a vital force minute to minute. No longer can a confidently successful secular society safely dismiss or ignore its religious fundamentalist members as "boobs," "know nothings" (H. L. Mencken), as "boosters," "yahoos," their minister-evangelists as "snake-oil salesmen," "Elmer Gantrys" (Sinclair Lewis). It is tempting to speak of the dissonance and atonality of the times, but this would mislead, I think, for it presupposes that there is *one* composition that is dissonant and atonal. What may be happening, actually, is the dissolution of one civil society into totally noncommunicating groups—a new sort of civil war. Former US president George W. Bush, reading his *Devotions for Morning and Evening* compiled by Oswald Chambers—a quickly digested paragraph per day—had no inkling perhaps of what another was reading in *Mother Jones* or *Foreign Policy* or in Immanuel Kant. The reverse was also true. It is hard for us to fathom and hold together the dissonance of rhythms in these everyday understandings.

Since my earliest references to Nietzsche in Segment 1, I have been developing the idea of the mind of music. It is now time that this idea reemerge focally. The best music is profoundly *adaptive* to the chancy world; it orients us as total bodily-mental-emotional beings. It is no accident, for example, that most symphonies are divided into four movements—constituting the "great form" as Robert Schumann put it. At many latitudes the seasons are four. The cardinal directions are four. We can also speak of the four ages of a typical human lifespan. The basic rhythms of all things are birth, growth, death, rebirth: timely effort, timely rest, timely joy and play, timely grief. In brief, great music orients us within the much-at-once, the chaos of life, which is not without pattern.

Some have argued that, roughly in the middle of the twentieth-century, music that falls within the classical tradition began to falter. If one accepts this, a plausible explanation suggests itself: It faltered because its ability to orient us within the much-at-once faltered. True, we get a cornucopia outpouring of kinds of music—blues, jazz, rock, country, all brimming with vitality. But what Nietzsche believed he found in the original Greek theater—the marvelous union of Dionysian and Apollonian ecstasies—is not vitally and reliably present. Vitiated are the peculiar reasoning powers, the Apollonian powers, of human minding (see Eugene Halton, *Bereft of Reason: On the Decline of Social Thought and Prospects for Its Renewal*, and also *Meaning and Modernity: Social Theory in the Pragmatic Attitude*).

Music commonly called classical had presumed to find some great form that could synopsize it all—could get it all in, all our minding, all our emotion. It is this presumption—it can be argued—that faltered at the midpoint of the last century. Recall in the previous Segment 7, when discussing the leaps beyond empirical verification taken by string theory in science, I suggested that great music analogizes this. Some passages of music analogize the empirical groundings and verifications of scientific activity. These are abuttings with directly evident, palpable bodily rhythms, approaches and recedings, postural and kinetic attitudes of our minding bodies. Other passages in music evoke the far-reaching swooping lines, targetings, speculations, and hypothesizing that are distinctively human. These are attempts at total orientation that have not yet been empirically verified.

Moreover, signature Native American thought and practice oversweeps and overlaps with all this. The point of their rituals and customs was to achieve through total activity a total orientation within the much-at-once. To be vitally invoked are the seven directions of the two-legged, upright animal's life. The four cardinal directions—north, east, south, west—plus the upper world where birds fly and see everything connected, and the lower world of earth, stable and empowering beneath our feet—these are the six directions—and the heart where everything is drawn together to feed and orient us is the seventh. What we might glimpse, sense, and hope for: a fellowship of science, music, art, living—a theory and practice of everything. To be sure, we remain comprehensive beings, and the impulse to comprehensive artistic activity is very strong. Great improvisational jazz, for example, taps into this desire for comprehensive inclusiveness:

> John Coltrane once said "the main thing a musician would like to do, is to give a picture to the listener of the many wonderful things he knows and senses in the universe." When Miles Davis asked him why he played so *long*, Coltrane answered, "It took that long to get it all in." (Danny Glover, Higher Ground Hurricane Relief Benefit)

Perhaps we would agree with the controversial notion that classical music began to falter in its vocation to orient us within the much-at-once around the midpoint of the last century. One might suggest that the much-at-once surges around us so abruptly, fragmentedly, and overwhelmingly today that music in the broad classical tradition simply cannot any longer manage to orient us within it, nor could any one type of music. The destruction that nations wreak is too astronomical to be comprehended even by the reason and mind of music. We are stunned—stunned literally—into artistic incapacitation, as if a bull had been led into the slaughter box and a massive sledgehammer had crashed down on its head. The bull falls uncannily quickly—like a bag of rocks.

The diabolical is the abruptly discontinuous. I once spoke with an elderly man who had been captain of a nuclear submarine during the Cuban missile crisis of October 1962. His craft was submerged in the North Sea.

It held sixteen nuclear-warhead missiles. He had to be prepared in five minutes to fire them at the Soviet Union. With the watery and translucent eyes peculiar to the very old, he said, "I was trained in World War II to destroy shipping, not to kill millions of people." Excluding psychopaths, is anyone today prepared to cope with a world that is beyond the human scale, that has so far outstripped our traditional frameworks of evaluation and orientation that we grope for any reason to do anything? Can we imagine it, millions of human lives snuffed out in a few seconds? The vast poisonous cloud, malignant beyond belief, drifting across Siberia, the Orient, the Pacific?

In the popular media we get a thudding emphasis on the Dionysian—shrieks, groans, grinds, or in country music and blues, laments and morose wailings. These may be strangely exciting, maybe moving. But do we feel guided and oriented when we are moved? In the original Greek music-drama, Dionysus shrieks when he is dismembered, torn to pieces (*sparagmos*), but in the greatest of the tragedies this dismemberment is in service to a reconstruction on a deeper and more abiding level of being human. Dionysus and Apollo are bonded. Within the classical music of the early half of the twentieth century, atonality pretty well finished its work when it became clear that it could do nothing else for us but realize our not-at-homeness.

No composer within the classical tradition has been more aware of the crisis than George Rochberg in his *The Aesthetics of Survival: A Composer's View of Twentieth-Century Music*. He writes that two key twentieth-century approaches to composition—the aleatoric (chance) technique and the rigidly controlled serial method—come out, ironically, sounding the same (*The Aesthetics of Survival*, 4). We have lost touch with what might be called the logic of the human bodily-self in the universe. Or, following Nietzsche, could we call it the mind of music? We must try to reclaim, Rochberg says, a "line of identity" running through music, holding it together because it holds together moments in actual human development that flower in realization or consummation. Or, perhaps, flower in the demise of human development, death, but it is the demise of just that—human development. Our bodily being, a resource for sounding the much-at-once, cannot long survive this extent of fragmentation.

Rochberg had first become known as a vehement practitioner of serial or twelve-tone music. Recall that this violent break with the "sentimentalism" and "clichés" of nineteenth-century music stipulated that no note on the row could be used again unless all the other notes had been used once. But catastrophic events in his life (he was seriously wounded in World War II and one of his children died) pushed him in a different direction. He felt impelled to write music with definitely human significance, returning to that deeper embodied sense resonant with the much-at-once and drawing forth a "line of identity." Composing twelve-tone music involved too much focus on solving puzzles, he came to feel, whereas the difficulties of life that are to be thematized in music are not just puzzles, not the outcome of abstract reasoning, but emerge from a felt sense. Note in his Symphony no. 2 (1955–56), after the screeching, the violation, the sound and the fury, some acceptance emerges, and, though maundering and grudging perhaps, some peace? At least the question is most intriguing. Human beings deeply need effort and restoration, struggle and consummation, potential and actualization—at least demonstrable failure. Lacking these rhythms that bring life into coherence, we grow stale, or crumble and fall to pieces, losing vital connection with the resounding much-at-once and its reverberations.

Rochberg's Symphony no. 5 (1984–85), first recorded in 2003 by the Saarbrücken Radio Symphony Orchestra conducted by Christopher Lyndon-Gee, is a talented, arresting, and gallant attempt to relocate that thread, that line of identity. It opens menacingly with slashing chords in full orchestra. The atonality—or better put perhaps, the bitonality—appropriately communicates the menace. Shocking, but is it shocking enough? Or too much so? The slow portion in the single-movement work is brooding and groping. It evolves into a kind of peroration that suggests to me William Faulkner's Nobel Prize speech, in which he claimed that "man shall prevail" in spite of everything—in the absence, one might imagine, of compelling reasons to think so. There is here a kind of Jamesian air that we must *think* so if we would possibly *do* so. It is an exhortation, not a thesis that might presently be proved: an exhortation to realign our abstract notions with the felt dynamic pulse of life. (Rochberg provides not only exhortations, but also consolations: Witness his beautiful *Transcendental Variations*, also recorded by the symphony on the same CD).

The question may be unfair, but I do ask: Do we actually feel centered, bolstered, prepared in the morning to "take on life"—as one radio therapist put it? All around us the much-at-once surges and boils, threatening diabolical annihilation. Where is that silence between waves, that Brucknerian peace, in which power is regathered regeneratively? Irene Klaver writes, "Silence is the resting place, where the attention given to words can evaporate. . . . Silence slips between representing something and being the something that is represented" ("Silent Wolves," 127). Which suggests the generative and regenerative center and ground of our being.

At times, I think, Rochberg's music does achieve the deeper layer of coherence and disclosure that Schopenhauer and Emerson named *reason* in contrast to *understanding*. This reason lies underneath words; sometimes it is a silence that lies between the representing and the represented, beneath the representational schema of the understanding alone. At points his music discloses what lies below consciousness—the unconscious domain in which the much-at-once permeates the body-self through and through, at the level of the life force, the *will* to live. Conveying it is a matter of *reason*.

In addition to the late Beethoven, we will always find some value in his earlier conquering spirit. But the heady confidence that the West must impose its values on the rest of the world is gradually being revised. We get a kind of lonely and eccentric Apollonianism that attempts to quarantine the Dionysian, to defy it when encountering it in other cultures, for example, in Islam. Apollo with his arrows—"far-arching Apollo" indeed! Self-satisfied brute strength and "rational" calculation will not be sufficient. Following Schopenhauer and Emerson, we need a much deeper conception of what *reason* is.

I think, with trepidation, that we need to be torn apart and reconstructed; we need that retreat of the waves in a turmoil of recuperation, the ominous pregnant silence between waves—which I am calling the Brucknerian peace. It is far from clear that we can achieve this, or that we even have the time or the will to try. It is far from clear what its musical counterpart would be today. In the very first pages of this book I wrote, "Music is the celebration, corroboration, enhancement, and support of the whole business of being human. It *authorizes* us to live fully." But we must ask now, at this more advanced point, whether it is even *possible* to generate this today.

Perhaps Philip Glass's music is another candidate for a viable contemporary classical music. With his signature repetitions, his arpeggios, he reinvokes vividly the power of ritual and trance. He supplies an obvious and, to many, a greatly welcome antidote to highly intellectualistic, disintegrative, abrupt and discontinuous classical music of the twentieth century. He touches on something primal in us bodily beings: repetitions, the very pulse of our identity. Glass prompts us to recall Nietzsche's praise of the primitive goat-man chorus in the Greek tragedies: their dithyrambic chanting and dancing in honor of Dionysus. Another avatar of this primal pulse is the chanting of Christian monks in the stone vaults of the cathedrals. We might think too of the pulses, the mysterious births, that open so many of Bruckner's symphonies, or to think of the pounding repetitions in his scherzos. But all these older examples of entrancement occurred in some well-established and deeply rooted setting: the whole tradition of Greek art and religion, or the Christian mysteries, or Bruckner's mystical Christianity, which is also a regenerative Nature mysticism. The absence of a well-rooted setting in Glass's music threatens his signature arpeggios with emptiness, aimlessness, and monotony, I think—at least when heard as pure sound in detachment from theatrical scene.

This prompts us to further clarify a distinction drawn earlier between trance and hypnotism. So far I've treated the distinction in a cursory and negative way, denying that the words can be used as synonyms and suggesting that trance exhibits varieties that hypnotism does not. But at this point much more can be made of the distinction. Hypnotism typically connotes a loss of autonomy, as one's present disposition is turned over to other agents and agencies, whereas beneficent trance—as I am concerned with it—is a matter of super-autonomy: It is what happens when genius is gripped by ecstasies of construction and imagination, by breakthroughs into novel ways of experiencing the world. True, I have spoken of genius caught up in countertrance, which supposes that one counters the deadening, routine, conformist trances of everyday life. I have also touched on Thomas Berry's critique of what he calls the technological trance. But now, in the music of Glass, do we get creative and constructive trance, or something more like hypnosis? I want to employ the terms more exactly.

It is no accident, I think, that Glass burst on the public scene in 1976 as composer for Robert Wilson's theater piece, *Einstein on the Beach.* Wilson is an eminently creative theater genius, and I suggest that Glass here found the setting that he needed for his music. In this theater piece we witness an attempt to guide and orient us within the much-at-once of our time. In a total work of art (also to the credit of Lucinda Childs's choreography and the scene designers), a dynamic and fluid Einsteinian universe was presented to us. We found ourselves liberated from the Newtonian box universe.

The curtains opened on the piece, disclosing the vast Metropolitan Opera stage nearly bare. Dominating the back of the stage was a huge, black-painted steam locomotive, apparently stationary, only its nose visible from the stage-left wings. A dancer spun slowly on the apron of the stage. With Glass's trancelike music sounding constantly, a voice was heard calmly intoning numbers. Joining this voice was a chorus of soft voices also intoning numbers. No connections between the voices, or between the numbers intoned by either source, could be detected. Then they were joined in a kind of trio by a woman's conversational voice, as if at a certain distance, though her specific words were not discernable. Evoked, perhaps, were the relativity physicist's matrix of numbers, mysterious to the layman. Although the locomotive was not visibly moving, one might have perceived that it advanced a little as the trio of voices gradually gave way to Glass's first extended stretch of locomotive music. Yet as the minutes—indeed hours—elapsed, it definitely could be seen to be traversing the stage. The tireless dancer moved in relentless diagonals, always moving backward toward the nose of the locomotive, facing us, inviting us somehow, then returning toward the audience—as if carrying some message to us.

The message became viscerally clear. With Glass's relentlessly pounding music, the huge locomotive is heard to move with tremendous inertia, but is not seen to do so at any particular moment. Traits that are locked together in the Newtonian box universe—locked together for the all-seeing eye of the alleged omniscient observer—are not presented together for mortal, finite, situated human experiencers, human witnesses. In the Newtonian view, the three dimensions of space, with their various spatial and temporal traits, are conceived visually as locked together in a container, which carries its contents inexorably along the track of time. In the Einsteinian view, we find a dynamic interplay of traits that are presented to, and are *relative* to, the human points at which they are experienced within the whole. The points count as individual to an extent that they could not within the Newtonian system of absolute space and absolute time. For Einstein, the fundamental unit is space-time, and reality is relative to its actual experienceability by finite observers.

While present at the performance, I felt all through my body the relativity of time and space, and how our being and identities are caught up within such a universe. I felt myself to be a participant, not just a presumptively detached observer. I felt we were *dreaming together* and had been drawn out into a place-time for slow, deep breathing—an oceanic experience—creating an astonishing line of identity. Reflecting later, I thought of Nietzsche. How did the Wilson-Glass-Childs production achieve this? How did it encompass to such a remarkable degree the uniquely eruptive and menacing much-at-once of today? First, the fact that we felt the much-at-once-encompassed allowed us to hold our attention upon it: We did not avert our attention in panic. Reminiscent of the strangely calming effect of Nietzsche's writing about the Greek theater, we felt that artists had cared enough for us to address us as we dangle in the abyss.

Some additional factors produced this achievement. The strange whole was assembled more like architecture than anything resembling a traditional opera, play, or cantata. That is, its development did not follow any traditional literary line—any dominance of well-crafted and well-venerated words. It did not follow any literary formula, whether romantic drama, adventure tale, or, say, Christian mystery or morality play. It was as unique as the much-at-once it was encompassing. How can we begin to grasp the astronomical scale of nuclear destruction possible within the Einsteinian universe? No mere blast of sound or blinding flash of light will quite do the trick. Largely due to Wilson's uncanny inventiveness, we heard the climactic episode of nuclear holocaust in renaissance-pure vocal lines, the blast of amplified instruments, a steady eighth-note pulse, and the now-hysterical chorus chanting numbers as quickly and frantically as possible (see the informative booklet accompanying the Elektra Nonesuch CDs).

With an expanded *reason*, we began to grasp numbers beyond comprehension. To cap the climax of artistic inventiveness, Wilson employed the services of a neurologically impaired boy, Christopher Knowles, in a short inserted play, "I Feel the Earth Move." Perhaps only with the help of the neurologically impaired can we begin to feel that the utterly taken-for-granted touchstone of stability, the earth, is now threatened with unparalleled alteration and disruption?

Older traditions of music-making gave us music to live with. It arrived with, and stayed with, its own abiding setting. The soundings of music go very deep, as well they should. Many people seem to have little trouble living with the experimentations and abstractions of twentieth and twenty-first century graphic and visual art; there, hanging on the wall as we converse happily in our living rooms, are Cubist works, or Mondrian structure and color abstractions, or Kandinsky pulverizations and explosions. The endemic detachment of visual experience allows us to live easily with these. But only disciplined experts can live with music in detachment—as something "out there" only. Try humming, say, an Alban Berg opera (*Lulu* or *Wozzeck)*. It does not sustain us in what must be the ever-ongoing structuring and maintaining of self.

Glass continues to develop his music today (a tenth symphony premiered in August 2012). Much of it is pure music with no palpable context in the world. He even dampens his signature arpeggios a bit. Some of it has a program; for instance, "The Dam," the third movement of his symphonic cantata *Itaipú* (1989), evokes the awesome monstrousness of the fifty-story-high, five-mile-wide dam on the Paraná River on the border of Brazil and Paraguay. To what effect does this piece sound in our world, caught up as it is in the technological trance? It isn't easy to say. The piece is exciting. But after the massed efforts and excitements, is the outcome regeneration or just exhaustion? It seems to me, mainly the latter. I don't find myself sustained in my autonomy. Glass sometimes speaks of his "portraits of Nature," but this suggests the limits of vision, not the depths of hearing, and of *reason*.

In Glass's Second Symphony (1994) we might hear "Brucknerian vistas" (James Jolly, *The Classical Good CD and DVD Guide*, 404), but the Brucknerian setting is missing. Gone is the regenerative cyclicity of Nature in the music, the inherently regenerative rhythms built into our bodies over untold millennia of evolution in Nature—particularly the Brucknerian moment when the waves recede back into themselves to regather their strength in silence or in relative quiet. It is not that there is no inventiveness in Glass. But instead of periodic consummation, relaxation, and dynamic maintenance of self, there is too often mere sounding, mere repetition—and in the end mere fragmentation, I'm afraid.

But of course, Bruckner's music is for all seasons and settings, and comparing most other styles of music to it is somewhat unfair to them. Composing on his deathbed in 1896, relativity physics was just around the corner. Yet as an expert organist and a renowned improviser on that instrument, Bruckner could also empathize with the sensibility of a medieval Christian in a vast cathedral. At the close of the nineteenth century, both in anticipation and recall, Bruckner placed the Newtonian mechanistic universe in question. That seventeenth-century physicist could write—and apparently mean—the universe is a machine, "but God is in the wheels thereof" (quoted in Wilshire, *Romanticism and Evolution: The Nineteenth Century*, 13). But what *could* it mean in terms of actual experience?

In a mechanical universe, all traits or characteristics are supposedly copresent, as we have noted, locked into place within their mechanical frame. But even light has a speed, and by the 1890s it was about to be precisely measured. Clearly, sound must travel and find us—and it will reverberate. It is true to say that as one of Bruckner's massive chords or chorales gives way to silence, it recedes into the past, but saying so is woefully incomplete. For the sound continues to resound in whatever way and to whatever extent the surroundings and our own body-minds promote. Moved and stanced in time—both in anticipation and recall—we must also be moved and stanced in space. So, viscerally experienced, Bruckner's music conveys the reality of space: the voluminousness of space extending in every direction all around us. His is the music of space, or rather of space-time.

This book is more cyclical than linear, as noted earlier, forming a progression in intensity. Conventional histories are linear: Events occur that seem to follow from the ones preceding. But of course the historians who recount these events cannot succeed in understanding their own lives in an exclusively linear way. They must exist, as we all must, in a kind of eternal present. One might call it a palimpsest: The past, the present, the future exist together, moving at their own velocities, yet appearing to us each moment as particles might suspended in a solution of liquid, as the now spreads before us predominating over other trajectories.

Consider the remarkable German-Russian composer Alfred Schnittke, who died in 1998, almost exactly a century after Bruckner. Schnittke conveys at least as successfully as Ives this sort of eternal present—the integrity of one's particular location within this vast unfolding of the world. It is an integrity embattled, I believe, beyond what Bruckner could imagine, one that must somehow defend itself against a scientistic-technological-totalitarian battering ram that defines the larger interplay of forces, and in the case of Schnittke's historical context, had given birth to the monster Stalin. Schnittke writes initially in the shadow of his revered Shostakovich, but he composes his own distinctive music. At his best Schnittke conveys what I have called the eternal present of each of our lives as we struggle to retain the integrity of who we are in a world dead set to flatten and absorb us in some rampage of acquisitiveness. This eternal present is not quite what Bruckner—that fairly devout Christian mystic—conveys, but it is deeply connected with it. Out of a blaring cacophony Schnittke very often peels away layer after layer of sound, as if he were seeking to penetrate these layers to reach a silence or a tone that had taken on the quiet solidity of silence. We are left with a background tone that is perceived as *having already been there* before we explicitly heard it. It is experienced as the abiding bass note, the stabilizing base note, of our being. Imperiled, yes, beleaguered, but not expunged. It must be close to what Christian mystics experience as God, or to what Emerson does.

Suddenly appearing in Schnittke are moments of heartbreaking nostalgia. Along with his sort of eternal present revealed, is the very ephemeralness of the present instant. In his *Stille Musik* for violin and cello (1979), when the strings are played dissonantly and often simultaneously, there sounds the essence of the tentative or the fragile—the just-was, the might-be, or the might-have-been. This reminds us that some human relationships (maybe even of oneself to oneself) never gel at all, never reach the cohesion of struggle, and so cannot entail any sort of resolution. The piece concludes with the episode of interaction of the two instruments going up in smoke. The violin rises upward in quiet glissando, ever thinner and higher, expiring in silence. The music puts us in mind of many of our incipient plannings, rehearsings, quasi-deliberations. These are real but evanescent. Nothing comes of these monologues; they pass, hardly leaving a trace it seems. This is music's mind, as Nietzsche put it, or music's reason, as Schopenhauer and Emerson write. Conveyed is *Wille*—will, life force—even if a *Wille* imperiled, embattled.

Schnittke's music can be called episodic, but it is a serious misjudgment, I think, to assert that his music is *only* fragmentary or episodic. After all, Bruckner's music might likewise be called episodic; he is reported to have said that before making a grand statement he must take a deep breath. Schnittke's music is very far from being composed of simple non-sequitors, discontinuities—like the word-salad of a schizophrenic—for this is the fragmentary and episodic rendered in art. The notes, written on the page, can be played, rendered again and again. It amounts to the episodic thematized, transformed, and in a sense transcended through being *composed* in art. Or, we can say, it is the episodic *rendered ritualistically.* (Incidentally, for evidence of Schnittke's reverence for Bruckner, consult a recording of his Symphony no. 2, *St Florian*—a symphony *cum* mass—with marvelous analytic notes by Alexander Ivashkin.)

Plato wrote in *The Statesman* that the wise ruler somehow manages to compare incomparables—apples and oranges, as we say—manages to deal with, to mensurate and measure, what are thought to be incommensurables. But all profoundly creative people do this. When Moshe Feldenkrais recognized the eyes as sphincters, for example, he did this; he saw and opened up the shocking and liberating consequences, as pointed out already. Schnittke in his musical sounds renders this dealing with incomparables.

Do Nietzsche's insights concerning the Greek theater long ago still really apply? There the performance was aimed at an audience that could recognize itself in the terms supplied by the dancing and chanting goat-men on the stage. The battering, shocking, apparently discontinuous events of everyday lives may be too horrifying to confront directly. But rendered effectively in art, they are encompassed and connected. Both Nietzsche and Schnittke are making this point. We might say that art supplies a *story* of the fragmentary and episodic, and that the storying in art has its own overarching continuity and coherence. There is some ecstatic surmounting, however hard-won it may be. Again, we encounter art's *reason* and *reasoning*—or *music's mind*.

It is often noted that we are the upright, bipedal, tool-using animal par excellence. This is greatly important. But something at least as important is not often noted: that we are the storytelling animal, and also the singing one—most primally, I think, when the story is sung. We *face* each other and communicate through many, many means. Imagine that we face each other in a circle around a fire and reinvoke—in a short time, linearly speaking—our whole lives together through time. We reinvoke an eternal present. Imagine ancient rituals in which things of unconditional value, of mythic importance, are reenacted again and again. Imagine how we hunter-gatherers held ourselves together through the bumps and shocks and traumas of time. Imagine how many of us today, torn from the past through a welter of eruptive events, caught up in our episodic and confused lives, can only encounter that eternal present through some kind of ritual performance, even if one shorn from God's Presence.

For many of us but not all, for never before has the United States been more splintered on the fundamentals of cultural-ritual life—and here I do not exclude the period of the Civil War. For many, the old mythic and religious verities do still hold. The sheer complexity of our more inclusive and intermixed society is necessarily more fragmented than any audience attending the ancient Athenian dramas could be imagined to be. Today the efficacy of the rituals still practiced in our experimental nation, as well as the default of newer shared rituals, must give us pause. Fundamentalists of all kinds tend to contract into small self-obsessed groups, and anyone who is critical of this whole way of thinking and being might call these clots in the arteries of an increasingly global world.

Let us try to achieve a still more sweeping and intensive gathering up of the themes of this book, which should also amount to new growth, a regenerative advance. We must try to weave identities, and we must do so in fugue-like ways within the much-at-once of the here and now. Our lives on our planet are changing so rapidly that the changes outrun the conceptual, the artistic, and, for many, the religious frameworks with which we must try to assess the meaning of what is happening. Traditions—traditions of interpretation—aren't just "nice to have" but are essential for being and becoming who we are.

The sciences make remarkable discoveries that contribute to this interpretive process.[1] Physiologists discovered the delicate yet strong muscles that expand and contract around the eyeballs, then Feldenkrais discerned them to be sphincters, connected organismically with the other sphincters in the body. Only then could he work out the profound implications for voluntarily healing the spasticities, hang-ups, disconnections in our living. Again, physiologists discovered peristaltic structures and functions: the peculiar wormlike wave motion of the intestines and other hollow muscular structures, produced by the successive contractions of the muscular fibers of their walls. Thus the explanation of how worms move was discovered, and scientific insight was gained into our own vital abdominal and intestinal structures.

Thousands of years ago Taoist thinkers and practitioners knew that the *dan tien*, which lies just beneath the navel within the body, was the energic source and taproot of the dynamic coordination of all the activities of body-self: It forms our core. But few people, particularly few "overachieving" Westerners, know of this tradition; though we have access to so many cultures today, it is a quite different matter to *inhabit* these traditions, as opposed to knowing of them as a curiosity. Nor do more than a

1. In the past several decades the scientific study of music on many fronts has amassed a considerable corpus. For only one example, see *Brain/Mind Bulletin* 10, nos. 4/5 (January 21 and February 11, 1985), which contains many worthwhile articles, but in particular see "Breaking the Code of Musicality," on the work of Manfred Clynes (republished in *Selected Papers (1972–1993) on Sentics and Manfred Clynes*, http://www.rebprotocol.net/senmanfredclynes2.pdf). When people experiencing particular feelings are asked to push a button, the graphs of "essentic" forms for each sort of emotion differ greatly. Two lines form a kind of graph for each emotion: love, hate, grief, joy, sex, anger, reverence, no emotion. The upper lines represent downward/upward pressure, the lower lines forward/backward pressure, while breaks in lines represent unevenness of pressure. According to the study, breaks in the lines occur most prominently in anger, grief, and hate; thus, scientific study coheres with ordinary perception, as in "trembling with anger, trembling with hatred." Music's meaning lies with the whole body in whole environments. Though the subjects may have been asked to remember or imagine experiencing their feelings, what they had to remember or imagine was experiencing these feelings *bodily* in particular concrete environments.

precious few grasp the revolutionary import of Western thinkers like Jean Gebser, who writes of the origins of consciousness in the convolutions and coils of the *intestines* (see Jean Gebser, *The Ever-Present Origin*). And yet the human need for integration and identity is so strong that attempts at assimilating these ancient physiological structures, still carried with us, show up in the arts. Nietzsche's goat-man chorus in ancient Greek drama immediately leaps to mind. I have explored, as well, Rochberg's and Schnittke's efforts of assimilation. What is the upshot of all this for our lives today in the twenty-first century?

So disruptively rapid is change that cultural traditions of interpretation are disabled, unavailable. This myriad of influences cannot be assimilated systematically, habitually, ritualistically into most people's daily lives. Identity building is not sustained. It is extraordinarily difficult to imagine the sort of genius required to lead us through the glittering debris. People who are "religious" in an established or traditional sense almost inevitably respond to the planet-wide cultural supermarket with grimace and aversion: It all so sensually indulgent and rootless. They are seeing something. But actually, taking the word "sensual" in a deeper sense—as the power of our senses to connect us with more potent dimensions of existence—it is not sensual enough. That is, the focus of our sensual awareness is not planted and oriented solidly on the earth and in our bony, muscular, nervy bodies. As Native Americans would say, we do not find our way confidently over the land day to day, year to year, generation to generation. In the concluding segment, the Final Benediction, I say more about the utterly essential role of well-grounded rituals in maintaining and empowering human beings. In this widespread, perilous, and turbulent much-at-once that holds, moves, and shakes us today, these rituals have never been more needed and have never been more difficult to achieve and to patiently cultivate.

FINAL BENEDICTION: RITUAL AS MUSIC

Every life is in many days, day after day.

—James Joyce

My wife and I and a close friend of many decades were aboard a ship looking for whales off the coast of California. After several hours of searching, we had found none. Finally we heard the captain's laconic voice announce, "Two humpbacks at 11 o'clock!" so we stamped out of the luxury cabin. There they were about fifty yards away: two vast, humped brown backs emerging from the sea and slipping back into it. The captain declared, "The largest is about forty-five feet long." As we got closer we saw the steam and spray issuing from their blowholes and heard their strange, hoarse, thunderous and primeval breathing. There was something peculiarly encompassing and pervading about this sound. Then, in an astonishing moment of realization, I became aware that *I* was breathing in synchrony with them. The hoarse, thunderous breathing was also my own! It issued rumbling not only from them, but from my own chest. For about forty minutes we followed the pair of animals, until it grew late in the day. On the way back to port, the guide observed, "They sleep with half their brain at a time."

For the first months of our very young lives we live in a watery world. It is crippling patriarchal prejudice to think that our reality begins at birth—that is, when each of us is separated from the mother. Our body's nervous system and osteomuscular structure was first formed and conditioned as we floated in amniotic fluid. We could not see, but we could hear. From every direction, when we were even upside down, the internal sounds of the mother interlaced with those of the fetus and with whatever booming or staccato or generally strange sounds penetrated the watery sack from the encompassing world. Our first environment was oceanic.

Of course, it is also true—momentously so—that we were born. Our first frantic gasp for air marked us. The world of air and separate palpable things found us. We soon learned the difference between upside down and right side up, between night and day, and could eventually stand upright and assume the life of the bipedal animal. We could take steps and stride and learn the meaning of linear time. We became a member of the species that distinguishes itself—for better or worse—from other species of living beings. So we must proceed most carefully in our account, identifying and distinguishing the different worlds of experience that successively formed us. But in our culture in particular it is easy to slip away from, to ignore, the watery world before birth.

We noted William James's key insight into the significance and power of music: that it can reinvoke the primal experience of the watery world, the oceanic feeling that is universal, that sends us ontological messages concerning our reality. As Schopenhauer and Emerson knew before James, these messages do not come in the form of *representations* of the world or of ourselves in it. They do not occur on the airy level of understanding merely. They are immediate, greatly potent, emotionally loaded disclosures or *presentations* of reality that move us. This is the *mind* and *reason* of music. If for some reason we are not moved, we are deficient in our *being.*

To be replete in our being, and truly functional, we must be capable both of receiving these ontological messages involuntarily and of reproducing some of them at will in our various arts, most obviously in music. First, allowing ourselves to be found by the world, then finding ourselves found in our arts. In this way the sacred all-togetherness of things, the Whole, gets woven into and through our voluntary careers. The earth's wilderness undergirds, infuses, and empowers us in our freedom. As with Black Elk during his first cure, the earth's energy can be felt to come up through our feet and into our legs to steady and steel us in resolve. That this steel can only emerge within the primal experience of the whole circumpressing cosmos, and out of our residual experience of the watery world, is certainly remarkable. Steel from water—a remarkable alchemy!

If these are indeed universal messages, as James insists, we should not be much surprised to find the Lakota shaman and warrior Black Elk and the contemporary Euro-American philosopher Henry Bugbee agreeing on a fundamental point: that it is song or anthem that conveys the deepest reality of our being; that these constitute the reason and mind of music, also the reason and mind of our selves. Mind is not immaterial but the fruit of the marvel and miracle of matter itself—matter and energy, whether light or dark. As Feldenkrais discovered, both the eyes and the anus are sphincters, and one depends upon the other and, indeed, all of us depend upon the All.

Recall that as Black Elk prepared during a stormy night for his first opportunity to cure, he heard the world all around him questioning him, asking for a reckoning. He listens intently to something, somewhere, somehow—something "all over the sky"—something that is everywhere and pluripotential. His response is to rise and sing the song of his great vision. We can connect this with Pythagoras of Samos who thousands of years ago wrote: The universe sings. We have noted key features of twentieth-century physics: nonlocality and superposition. Things are not simply located and sealed off from other things; they are not sealed up within their own surfaces. Things once together at their source remain in instantaneous resonance when far apart. We also noted string theory in physics and putative harmonies and synchronicities between these incredibly tiny vibrating strings. In this vein Bugbee wrote, "as true stillness comes upon us, we hear, we hear" (*The Inward Morning: A Philosophical Exploration in Journal Form*, 221), clearly implying that we hear more than we can say, as Black Elk also believed, certainly more than we can say in any literal prosaic speech or writing. Only the music of words, poetry, or words-and-music—an anthem that discloses us to ourselves and others—only these modes of *reason* have any chance of disclosing what is meant.

These messages retained in music from the watery world of gestation, just as "waters of the infinite ocean send their waves to break among the pebbles that lie upon our shores" (James, *The Varieties of Religious Experience*, lecture 9, 334)—don't these messages deliver to us, signed and sealed, a redemptive unity or unification with the All? Caught up in some ecstatic moment we may slide into this affirmation! It is sorely tempting to believe this. We so desire to believe this. But it would be a terrible error to believe so. The error would be egregious because, as Charles Peirce put it, it poisons the well: It generates, flows, pools into countless other errors. It masks out the other fundamental dimension of our being: that we *are* born, that we emerge into the pedestrian, quotidian world of air, our daily stepping linear life, the world of things and moments that are—for our inescapably practical selves concerned with survival—separate enough, formidable enough. It would mask out that we are birthed into *this* quotidian life, and would mask out the masking out, leading to a pathetic and dangerous ignorance.

I have already alluded to the pivotal role played by Gustav Mahler in the history of music and civilization. He composes on the cusp where conventional tonal music of the nineteenth century leads into the atonal world of the twentieth. Another way of putting this: on the cusp where the assurance of resolution and repose within the sacred all-togetherness of things becomes very blurred, ambiguous, uncertain. It is no accident, I think, that sounds of water emerge at crucial points in his major compositions: His musical tones flow into, directly abut within, the watery sounds of life that they convey. In this great swirling mass of watery sound, it's easy to imagine a large oar driven down energetically into the mass, stirring it, and even to imagine oneself submerged, caught in the vortex, gasping for air.

Thus propelled by massed tones at its opening—thrusting forward as if by a great oar—is his Symphony no. 7 in E Minor, *Song of the Night*. Water sounds also at crucial points in what is arguably Mahler's first completely mature composition, his Symphony no. 3 (the one that "floats your teeth," as musicologist Jack Diether once observed to me, impatient with my unresponsiveness at that point in my life). But I want to focus on its use in the Symphony no. 6 in A Minor (*Tragic*), the one that, during rehearsals, frightened Mahler himself. There are literally three hammer blows in its fourth and final movement. Mahler called for a large wooden mallet like a sledgehammer to be swung down on a large block of wood.

He wanted his musical tones to consummate themselves in the very *sounds* of matter being struck. Walking at night once in the cobblestone square outside the great Cologne cathedral, a person walking next to me fell suddenly and struck his head on the stones; I think this is close to the sound that Mahler wanted. (None of the performances I have heard, live or recorded, have followed his directions—I don't know why—though in a fine recorded performance by George Szell and the Cleveland orchestra, a bass drum is struck sharply instead.)

After a blow has been struck, there occurs this vast swirling watery sound, very much as if someone has been struck on the head, submerged in water, but still paws and kicks his way to the surface. Then a resolute marching occurs, a retaining of the previous marching motif in the symphony. This continues almost to the point of an ultimate weariness, then a second blow is struck. The first blow's aftermath is repeated. Then more marching sounds, then a third blow. Again there is the swirling of water, but weaker, and a dying out in the symphony follows. But it will not end on this failing and falling away. A terrible burst of full orchestra finishes off the symphony—and the poor suffering being whom we imagine. Or is this a final burst of defiance from him? In any case, silence falls.

The movement of these great watery tones evokes not just a dizziness and imbalance but a vivid sense of pluripotentiality. This word from embryology, which I have applied to Black Elk's experiencing in the night's stormy wilderness before he is to face the sick boy, seems clearly to apply to this swirling, churning music. What will come of the event? Indefinitely many things could follow. One thinks of Peirce's notion of chance. Then of Nietzsche's writing of awful accidents. The possibility of a demonic or diabolical response, closing off the openness of the cosmos in a person's experience. A bitter, obsessive defiance, with clenched teeth? Any grief, say, that cannot be mourned through will leave the sufferer fixated, stuck, unable to pass on to something new. We might be reminded of Arrigo Boito's second opera *Nerone* (Nero): the dreadfully rapid treading passage, peg-legged treading that is faster than humanly possible. We don't get the superhuman here, only the diabolical. There are untold numbers of instances of this diabolism—within and outside the arts.

It was just chance that I happened to be walking close to the fellow who fell and struck his head on the stones in Cologne that night. That sound will always be with me. Yet Schelling is right to remind us that chance is not only inescapable, but that it is the site of our freedom also. I am always free to reconfigure, reframe, recontextualize the event. If I *realize* this, I remain open in an open cosmos. I am not locked into the false infinite of diabolical rage or sadness—that little speck of white infection, as Kierkegaard pointed out, on the kernel of the grain. The sources of illumination can never be completely illuminated, Schelling makes this clear in *The Ages of the World*. Thinking that a few moments of oceanic feeling is redemptive is an insidious form of self-deception and diabolism, for masked out is the dailyness of living and, as I've pointed out, the masking out of the masking out. We forget our grave need for what the Lakota people identified as the "cold wind of the North that teaches endurance": our need for life-sustaining rituals that hold life together from one moment to the next.

In this Final Benediction I point to some life-sustaining modes of therapy that can function as de facto rituals, introducing something that is sorely lacking among many completely secularized people today. They also function as de facto ways in which we can become our own chorus—referring again to ancient Greek theater. This is so because those involved typically agree on what is happening and constitute a consensus on this. Released from a too-close attention to ourselves alone—too close to really see ourselves as minding-bodies-in-the-world—we join a *being*-building consensus as to who and what we are. For, of all the remarkable features of hurtling, bustling, often frantic contemporary life, perhaps the most remarkable deficit is this: the disintegration of traditional ritual for many secularized people. Life has always been a daily matter, renewing itself day after day. How to hold life together—on the individual and group levels—given the bumps and crises and disconnects that routinely happen?

Traditional societies addressed this need *to be* with rituals. These were synchronized and attuned with the great cusps, pivots, turning points of the seasons of the year and the individual lifecycle, as if by being so attuned the inexorable course and force of the wheeling year would carry the ritual observants through rough patches of time, predictable and unpredictable pits and black holes that can open and swallow us. Take, for example, the basal role of music in particularly pivotal rituals: *rites of pas-*

sage, in which adolescents are conducted from youth to adulthood. This is often the most precarious time in an individual's growth. Adults must supervise the passage: Children alone cannot raise children during this period. Adults must set the course of the passage to be traversed, evaluate the success or failure of initiates, and greet successful candidates when they reach the other side—adulthood.

Consider two very different rites of passage with startling similarities of aim: initiation into adulthood as practiced in an African culture (see Malidoma Patrice Some, *Of Water and the Spirit*), and on the other hand, the well-known bar mitzvahs and bat mitzvahs practiced by Jews in North Atlantic culture and around the world. In the African rite, the role of drums and incantatory soundings at various stages of the initiation is prominent. In the case of Jews, songs may be sung to punctuate the proceedings. Both groups of initiates must prove themselves capable of adult achievements. The Africans must endure prolonged physical hardships and achieve various vision quests in mountainous or jungle areas. The Jews must, among other things, show themselves capable of reading the difficult Hebrew language and reciting it from the sacred scriptures intelligently.

In both the African and Jewish rites, the celebrations that finally follow successful initiation are tumultuous and marvelous: various participatory entertainments, dancing, singing, feasting, drumming, and so on. When they have successfully traversed the passage, the initiates *know* that they are adults! The rootlessness and waywardness of too many secular youths today is appalling. There has occurred quietly and insidiously all around us a breakdown in the formation of human reality. Our forms of access to and articulations of the much-at-once, by channeling its power into activities and distractions that are suffocating and corrosive, have distorted its regenerative capacity. In the preceding segment I touched on the possibility that classical music has been overwhelmed today by mainstream culture's denatured manifestations of the much-at-once.

In Part I, I alluded to the marvelous W. B. Yeats poem that ends, "And shout a secret to the stone," and made bold to tell the secret. It is that we experience intimate affinity even with mineral beings—or can do so if our instincts have not been badly injured by too much city life and "civilization," as John Muir put it. Our bones are living minerals, the scaffolding that holds together ligaments, nervous and glandular systems, muscles, organs, flesh and blood, so that we can be *one* being maintaining itself through time. Our bones vibrate with whatever influences, disturbances, impulses occur: They are the ground base in a harmony, providing the bass note of reality that may never properly be acknowledged, never reach the articulable focus of awareness.

There is a knowing effected by the trunk, the ribcage, the backbone and sternum, the glands, the whole business. All feelings and behavioral tendencies involve this portion of the body. It is here that linear time may—just may—lose its disintegrating and alienating effects, as there is an unfolding of capacities in our bodies to sound the much-at-once. As we have frequently noted, much traditional European thought is vision-dominated. Vision is the distancing and detaching sense without equal. Given the ensemble reality of the senses, vision is anticipatory touch—*anticipatory* because implicit in our seeing is an incipient sense of the time it would take to reach the thing seen, if we should try to reach it. One can say that this also applies to hearing, though not as baldly or boldly, for hearing tends to be much more involving emotionally with the whole surround.

But when we know with our whole kinesthetic and proprioceptive bodily selves, there need be no distance between experiencing and what is experienced, no sense of the time to be traversed if we should try to touch the thing experienced. Differently put, there is no representation distinct from something represented. Even with hearing, it may take time to cock the ears and locate the source of the sound. The trunk of the body, on the other hand, is fairly nondirectional: It is not "on the way"; it is *already with* that to which it resonates. In our trunks we are *representing* nothing. We simply *are.* We exist within that *presence.* Again, we are living on the level of *reason*—properly grasped—not merely of *understanding.*

Of notable therapies, let us first consider Eugene Gendlin's therapeutic method called *focusing.* Our powers of cerebral absorption in abstractions tend to leave the rest of our bodies in oblivion. The discipline of focusing entails attending to the whole body's nascent and primal tendencies to sustained and regenerative living, allowing them to reveal themselves, preventing them from being squelched, nipped in the bud. The point is to give the whole body permission and encouragement to be what it deeply wants and needs to be, formed as it was in hunter-gatherer ambiences, contending with challenges and liberties over many millennia. Gendlin lets us in on one of his techniques:

> When people say something that they deeply mean, we can ask: "If the word/phrase __________ could mean just exactly what you wanted it to mean . . . [slight pause, change in tone, very gently continue]
>
> . . . what
>
> would
>
> you want
>
> it to mean?"
>
> ("Introduction to 'Thinking at the Edge,'" 1)

The gentle falling and softening of the voice has a patent musical quality. I think that Gendlin puts his finger on a far-ranging musical truth that is simultaneously a truth of our spiritual-bodily being. I now think I understand why certain cadences of music that fall gently by half-steps have always magnetized me; for example, the toccata of Bach's Toccata and Fugue in F Major (BWV 540) or the central cadence in the first movement of Mozart's *Prague Symphony* (Symphony no. 38 in D Major, K. 504). It is what Christians would perhaps call the grace of God, or people not so lofty in their ideology would viscerally recall in hidden memories of being picked up and comforted when, as infants, they cried out in desperation and helplessness. It is grace that acknowledges our neediness and answers it. The truth shall make us free, said Jesus, but it must be reaffirmed ritualistically.

In this passage Gendlin introduces us to his general scheme of things:

> "Thinking at the Edge" . . . is a systematic way to articulate in new terms something that needs to be said but is at first only an inchoate "bodily sense." . . . Whereas everywhere else in the university only

> what was clear counted at all, here we cared only about was as yet unclear. If it was clear I said "We don't need you for this; we have it in the library already." . . . All educated people "know" such things in their field of study . . . but typically people assume that it "makes no sense" and cannot be said or thought into. . . . "Oh," one student exclaimed when he grasped what I was looking for, "you mean something about which we have to do hemming and hawing?" "Yes, that was just what I meant." Another asked: "Do you mean that crawly thing?" ("Introduction to 'Thinking at the Edge,'" 1)

Gendlin builds on primal insights achieved by James, Peirce, Dewey, Heidegger—and also the American writer Willa Cather. To equate mind and consciousness, as Descartes did, is a dreadful mistake. Before we find or discover anything truly important, we have already been found. Our first task is to remain open to this vibratory ambience or tendency, this crawly thing that already enwraps us outside the articulable focus of everyday talking consciousness. As James wrote, at long last, we must do justice to the vague. There are no guarantees. If we always demand them, we will remove ourselves from the fecundity of the universe, the curious sense of the whole cosmos, which in its unfolding is enfolded within the present much-at-once, and which, in its own time, locates and finds us in our very frequent lostness.

Let's look now at a different therapeutic method, one with a coincidence of aim. It is called *tapping*, and recalls the use of drums by Native Americans, and indeed the percussive use of the whole body by African Americans. Seldom do ostensibly liberating thoughts and statements truly liberate, for they are disengaged from the whole body and leave it unaffected in its neuromuscular and glandular depths, visceral complexities, and bony resonances. The body is left unsupported in its dailyness. Tapping is a way of almost literally drilling liberating statements into the body and molding new behavior. It attacks headlong the cemented polar opposition: mind over against body. There are portions of the body closely associated with flows of energy (*chi*) that Chinese medicine has long identified and used, for example, in acupuncture. Tapping is a matter of systematically and rhythmically tapping or percussing in sequence these areas of the body. At the first area one utters a description of one's state of feeling; then, at the next, one utters an affirmation. For example, one's description might be: *Even though I feel helplessly angry at everything . . .* One's affirmation might be: *I choose to find new and refreshing ways of coping with anger.* Or it might be: *I nevertheless fully and completely accept myself.* To tap the body is literally to tap the core of our feelings, to play upon our bodies as the musical instruments of our felt sense in the whole.

This recalls Nietzsche's aphorism: Of everything that happened to me, to be able to say "thus I willed it" (*Thus Spoke Zarathustra*, "On Redemption," 139). In a regenerative rhythm, a wise receptivity, one first allows oneself to recognize how one has already been found affectively by the world. Then one actively asserts one's affirmation, which will probably lead to another wise receptivity and yet another affirmation, and so on. When one finds a cadence and a response that works, that clicks, one repeats it ritualistically—not just when it is immediately needed, but also sometimes when it doesn't seem to be needed at all. Life is many days, day after day.

Someone might object, "This is only because you believe both statements; it is merely an act of ephemeral autosuggestion." But the practice of tapping needn't have merely passing effectiveness. It directly confirms the distinction that Schopenhauer and Emerson drew between mere understanding and primal reason. To be effective, some practitioners maintain, one needn't believe that the statements are true or sincere. One simply repeats them while tapping, one "goes through the motions," and nonetheless as one speaks, the whole body, the whole body-self thinks, rhythmically moves, effectively resolves on some prereflective, preverbal level—though I am inclined to think the therapy is more effective when one asserts the affirmation feelingly and believingly. This *reason* is not abstract reason but rather a deeper level of "happening" attuned with the whole that we can literally tap into.

That a practice such as tapping should be needed, and that it is effective, is astonishing but plainly true, I believe. To cobble together hyphenated terms—mind-body, body-self—and to think that this alone does the job of integrating the self is only verbal evasion and self-deception. We need to grope our way to methods for actually and deeply integrating our animality-humanity day after day. We need to find ways of reenacting Nietzsche's chorus of goat-men circling and dancing around the solo characters on the stage. We need to find ways of perceptively and humbly—humanely and artfully—accepting our animality. Perhaps too, if we listened to a bird and heard it as the sounding of an evolved dinosaur, we would plumb and stretch our deep memory, and thereby plumb, stretch, and integrate ourselves. Might we *plume* ourselves? We need the deepest of rituals. We can think of tapping as tuning ourselves: Becoming ecstatically attuned to ourselves in the Whole, we are filled and sustained. But, of course, we must be prepared to do it ritualistically.

A third method with a coincidence of aim that is still highly distinctive—aimed at integration of self into cohesive and satisfying abiding and agency—is Alexander Lowen's *bioenergetics* (I am indebted to Laura Melling for this discussion). Lowen's definition of health, which complements an implicit theory of democratic social organization, is of a balanced dynamism between bottom-up and top-down energies. As most Westerners feel disconnected from their feet and legs, much of bioenergetic therapy consists in grounding practices that promote the flow of bodily energy upward from the ground. Lowen compares the exercises to Tai Chi, but stresses the difference: the latter ancient practice assumes that practitioners have no major body disturbances, whereas this is not the case for most Westerners. We must work out the tensions built up in our bodies by chronic defensive holding patterns before we can properly align ourselves to universal harmonies in movement meditations; these defensive patterns are sometimes, for example, a holding onto demonizing others different from or alien to us, yet we end up carrying them around with us as blockages in our bodies. Chronic defensive holding patterns very probably involve cramped and tightened sphincters—including the squinting of the eyes.

We can't help but recall Black Elk's experience during his first cure when the sick boy smiles at him; the healer, feeling reassured, experiences energy coming up through his legs from Mother Earth. We are the creatures who feed on the six directions, who can be grateful for the gifts from each, who can allow ourselves to be found and to be gifted at our hearts—our chests and abdominal centers—which is the seventh direction. This beneficent undergoing is the dark and fertile seedbed or seminarium for regenerative initiatives, activities, creations, re-creations. It is the seedbed for our *being*.

Clearly, all these therapies aim to rejoin us with our own body-selves as these have been formed over countless generations through creative adaptation to wilderness environments. I supply a final example from my own hard-won experience of therapy. About twenty years ago, unhappy with my life and my workaholic intellectualism, I submitted myself to a health practitioner who had trained under Ida Rolf. That pioneering body worker had developed a way of addressing fixations and negative feelings locked in the muscles of the body and quite impervious to "more civilized" talk therapy. Her method consisted in breaking down with her hands the tensed sheathing or fascia enclosing and trapping the muscles. At times the Rolfian treatment is painful. The final session in my series involved cranial osteopathy, or working on the muscles of the face and head, which capped things off (pun intended). The very last intervention—you are forewarned about possible queasiness—entailed the practitioner's inserting the well-lubricated little finger of her gloved hand into my nostrils. From there she gently probed the sinus cavities, insofar as she could do so. With the first probe I heard a strange, high-pitched voice say, "Momma!" It was my own voice!

To offer a bit of background, some years previously I'd had the extraordinarily odd experience of—how else to describe it?—feeling my father's body moving inside my own. It was not a *sign* of my father's walk or a *representation* of this. It was not the work of mere understanding but of *reason* in Schopenhauer's and Emerson's startling sense of the term. My father's walking body presented itself within my own and occupied it. This was the most immediate of all possible experiences of immediacy. It did not represent something not itself. I was elated. It was as if one of Emerson's "auxiliaries," or what Greeks and Romans had called tutelary spirits, had spontaneously come to help me. I participated in a life force—*Wille*—that was beneficially communal.

I had similar experiences with my aunt, who had helped raise me during the years of the Great Depression. Her body, in some of her moments, had been absorbed into mine. Occasional flashes of my grandparents also occurred. But never before this time had I found my mother absorbed in my entrained body. I suppose she had always been there somehow—but as yet unaccessed. Too painful, too disturbing? I don't know. I'm still developing my relationship to her. Fortunately at the time of this writing, she still lives and is lucid at a hundred four years old, and I can attempt to trace the murky, intricate, and utterly basic relationship of absorption in her. The first clue, as I said, was the sound of my own voice crying "Momma." I don't believe at all that this was or is demonic or diabolical. Just the opposite. It cleared a blockage and opened me up to my immediate source in the cosmos, my mother, hence to the cosmos itself. The basal watery level, the pluripotential, emerged in this form, and it was and is very good. In those moments I felt that I was falling in love with the cosmos (see the writings of American philosopher Josiah Royce).

But what hope is there for *humanity*? Only a few persons have the resources—of whatever sort—to engage in these modes of therapy. What can we say except that it is up to each of us to really awaken ourselves and look about in those moments when we realize that we otherwise live mainly asleep. Then we can hope that this wakefulness might spread, that many others will realize that what binds us together as human beings is more fundamental than what divides us. We share the earth and our bodily beings and our origin in the cosmos. We also share, of course, our desperate need for sustenance moment to moment. We need water, we need air—that for which we gasp particularly desperately in certain moments. We trace our way reliably to the whole only through our immediate origins, our own parents.

I think it is up to each of us to find and hear that anthem that is our own voice, or rather, to let it find us. The self calls to itself. We hear Bugbee's chant yet again:

> As true stillness comes upon us, we hear, we hear, and we learn that our whole lives may have the character of finding that anthem which would be native to our own tongue, and which can be the true answer for each of us to the questioning, the calling, the demand for ultimate reckoning which devolves upon us. (*The Inward Morning*, 221)

Might we choose to regard this final repetition of the chant on these pages as the *benediction* that rounds out and completes this book? *Bene-diction* in its root meaning evokes good-saying, the saying of goodness. Not a saying about goodness, not a representation of it, but a presenting of it, its presence resonating within us, an evocation of it in its power. What if we believed that this presence will evoke previous evocations and anticipate future ones? What if we endured in the resolve to reinvoke such a presence ritualistically? I think this could very well be the weaving of fugal strands that holds us together ecstatically through time.

APPENDIXES

APPENDIX A

MORE ON FUGUE, MIND, AND THE SELF

As I've argued, the fugue is an immensely attractive musical form because it conveys the essence of self to oneself: the weaving of self through time by retrieving what it has previously done and projecting what it might do. Or, put another way, the fugue conveys the self to itself by *returning* itself to itself, and in so doing the self defines, excites, augments, and emboldens itself. Returning ourselves to ourselves in all our fugal density and complexity, we might extrapolate and catch an inkling that there is more to one's self than one can be aware of. This need not disconcert us; to the contrary, it can anchor our awareness of our reality. As both Edmund Husserl and William James note, when something presents itself as actual and not fictional, it presents itself as more than can ever completely appear, more than can ever be grasped.

James wrote in 1905 that the body, typically present on the margins of awareness and "peculiarly warm," is the abiding "storm center of all this stress" through time ("The Experience of Activity," 211n1). Thanks to rapidly developing means of imaging the brain, scientists can trace how all activity we deem "mental" involves not only the cerebral cortex but also the brain's thalamus and motor cortex, hence all "mental activity" is also bodily and brain movement, overt or incipient (see Rodolpho Llinás's notable *I of the Vortex: From Neurons to Self*).

Mammalian selves are more or less elaborated. A distinction occurs in mammalian organisms between what they do and what all other things do; they move voluntarily while most other things remain comparatively stationary, for instance. Thus a rudimentary self first appears: The organism-self feels itself abiding-in-its-own-places—not necessarily with *words*. Hence, for these places to be habitually disrupted or expropriated by others is for this organism-self to be traumatized. In elementary proprioception, organisms locate their own bodies, the disposition of their limbs, and so on; they are thus set off from everything else in the cosmos. Even with those mammalian organisms that pass the "mirror test" for primordial selfhood, some of this proprioceptive activity probably never reaches even the margins of their awareness. In the "higher" nonhuman mammals, is there ever an awareness of the awareness, some primordial awareness of self-as-aware, an awareness that the awareness is "mine"? I wouldn't know how to test for this, so must assume that my question is moot.

There is continuity, presumably, between human and nonhuman organisms. Hence much of the human self must lie outside awareness, though much of what lies within it seems to be distinctive to our species, and is sometimes disturbing to ourselves. In human mammals, proprioceptive activity that reaches some sector of awareness can sometimes be recognized as "my" awareness. We not only use signs, often well aware that we use them, but we can become absolutely fascinated and carried away by them—even to the point of concealing or distorting portions of our own mental life, as already noted. Hence my particular interest in that fugal variation on the theme called "inversion." How do we conceal something of ourselves *from* ourselves? One chief way is by coding or signing it as *not to be signed, noticed, or recognized further.* Thus the trick of self-deception is accomplished. We conceal ourselves and conceal the concealment from ourselves. We drop into ho-hum trance.

Implicit in the dynamic fugal structure of the self is that, in perpetually retrieving itself, the self must also perpetually "throw itself before itself," must judge and evaluate itself—in this respect being the opposite of trance—or else it must deliberately evade responsibility for doing so. In either case, responsibility remains to be either accepted or evaded. As Schelling put it, we never escape the site of our freedom. In the end, not to accept responsibility for one's actions is not to be a full or authentic human self.

So we should not be surprised that when notable composers approach the end times of their lives they crave a summing up of themselves—an "ultimate reckoning that devolves upon us," as Henry Bugbee put it well (*The Inward Morning*, 221). It is no accident that while he approached death, J. S. Bach worked on *The Art of the Fugue* (BWV 1040), in which he exhibited many of the forms it could take. The last example breaks off and hangs in the air—unfinished. Death intervenes, unforgettably. But unforgettable also is the self's articulation and assertion of itself in the face of the utmost peril. It is a remarkable elaboration of the animal instinct to continue in existence, to survive. One *might* argue—though I would not—that this is a noble form of self-deception, being presented with responsibility in such a way that one cannot follow up on its intimations; but rather than being a failure of authenticity, I think, it is a sublime form of it.

A further example is the last major work of Danish composer Carl Nielsen entitled *Commotio* (op. 58, 1931), a set of two complex fugues for organ, interlinked subtly. *Commotio* would be literally translated into English as "commotion," but what Nielsen actually means is far different: It is that motion or movement in which the self reflects, explores, and expands itself in order to evaluate itself. Nielsen planned to take the composition from Denmark to Lübeck on the Baltic Sea for a first performance. But again, death intervened. He got there only in the sense of spiritual-animal protention and anticipation.

Also in this vein, I've noted Bruckner's attempts on his deathbed to complete the final movement of his last symphony. According to Austrian conductor Nikolaus Harnoncourt, the composer projected a review of the leading themes of his earlier symphonies. He also began to sketch an extraordinarily complex fugue that would shrink in midflight from four to three bars. He was challenging himself, taking his own measure, seeking a superior form of his self's life. Could we say that he was seeking to unpack his soul?

Here it would be strangely remiss not to mention the final movement of Mozart's last symphony (Symphony no. 41 in C Major, K 551, *Jupiter*), a majestic five-part fugue, or inverted quintuple counterpoint. It was created at a very bad time in his short life marked by illness, black thoughts, creditors badgering him, his life moving toward death. Perversely and maddeningly enough, although he was celebrated throughout Europe, no court position was offered him. His last three symphonies were composed in less than three months. William Molloch writes, "He wrote the symphonies for some unknown purpose, perhaps out of sheer desperation" (notes to Symphony no. 39, Telarc CD; see the superb recordings by the Prague Chamber Orchestra, with Sir Charles Mackerras conducting). Writing to a friend about composing some dances to keep food on the table, Mozart remarked, "This is what I do, not what I can do." Sigmund Freud seems to be right: What we have in the end is just love and work. It is that which pours itself into a fugue, as one comes home to oneself and to the cosmos that parents one.

As noted in Segment 2, a fugue is self-compounding. It conveys and reinforces the self's attempt to get a grip on itself, to take initiatives in its choices, and to hold itself responsible. Though death is the main challenge to us human organisms, it is certainly far from being the only one. We are porous and emotional beings, easily hurt, who try to protect ourselves. Along with religion, music aims to heal and comfort us—*religio medici.* English composer William Walton's First Symphony (Symphony no. 1 in B-flat Minor, 1935) emerged from a greatly troubled time in his life: A romantic relationship had given way and landed him on the rocks. In composing, he tried to deal with his anger—rage, really—and his hurt. He relied on music for the truth. His direction for the symphony's scherzo is delicious—*con malizia*—with malice. The symphony's first three movements were given a full-scale orchestral performance, but he found himself incapable of completing the fourth and final movement for a considerable time and it may have seemed to him unfinishable. Finally though, it emerged, leveraged itself into being, turning and twisting itself. It held a fugue at its core.

Another example is Benjamin Britten's *Prelude and Fugue for 18 Strings* (op. 29, 1943): A doleful, dragging, tormented introduction is shouldered aside by an effervescing, frothing, rollicking fugue. A revealing conveyance, it seems to me, of the reality of freedom, spontaneity, potentiality, and the power of individual decision and agency, recalling William James's words on freedom: "Yes, I can!"—"Yes, I can!" (see Victor Kestenbaum, *The Grace and the Severity of the Ideal: John Dewey and the Transcendent*). By tapping into the resources of our mammalian species and its individual members, the self partakes of the reality of the sacred. As musicologist Alfred Einstein says of Mozart's development as a symphonist, he moves from the merely "external" and "ceremonial" to "spiritual avowal" (*Mozart: His Character, His Work*, 216).

Sometimes a self returns to itself in anticipation of and commitment to what it will do in vivid obviousness: a vowing in which the whole body-self generates the vow. Thus athletes may vividly rehearse in sequences of total bodily imagery or schemas what they are about to do. As in pole vaulting: Standing poised on the runway, vaulters anticipate the moves, motions, steps and turns they will take to create the ideal vault, and this "running through" is actually a vowing to do just these anticipated things. Athletes perpetually feed these back into themselves, as selves who vow, and this vowing may make the difference between success and failure in executing the vault. This is a self-compounding, self-creating process. One ecstatically holds oneself capable and responsible and is thereby balanced, righted, stayed, empowered.

To expect little of oneself is to lack the severity and grace of the ideal. Comfort and convenience reveal themselves as false ideals that put one out of touch with the reality of one's potentiality. It is to remain suborned to our species' protracted period of dependency: our need for support and recognition by caregivers. One slides into the entranced and infantile delusion that just to be recognized by others—say a mob of adoring fans—is to be stayed, solid, and sound. But the truth is that sometimes we must endure alone and take leaps in the cold, unsure whether they will succeed. We thereby test and confirm our reality. Part of the severity of the ideal is avoiding being drawn into false ideals in which the scope of one's powers of anticipation and identification shrink. One becomes absorbed in the merely parochial, in the obviously "exciting," or in short-term ecstasy. In a desperate bid to avoid boredom, one repeats what one is doing, real freedom is gone, and trance or addiction has one in its clutches.

APPENDIX B

CAN BRAIN SCIENCE TELL US WHO WE ARE?

In the preface to *Musicophilia: Tales of Music and the Brain*, Oliver Sacks sagely writes, "These new insights of neuroscience are exciting beyond measure, but there is always a certain danger that the simple art of observation may be lost, that clinical description may become perfunctory, and the richness of the human context ignored" (xiv). He goes on to write that both brain science and the "simple art of observation" are necessary. But here we should explore why both are necessary. Studies of music and the brain interdigitate and interweave; the very obviousness of it may trigger the unwarranted inference that brain science alone can tell us who we are. To evoke one of indefinitely many possible examples, the first movement of Mozart's Symphony no. 31 in D Major, K 297, *Paris*, exhibits a descending passage in full orchestra in which three steps of the fulsome descent interweave regularly and normatively with one sound of a singular set of instruments. This interweaving of rhythms forms a master metarhythm that bewitches, magnetizes, and delights attention, as if we could sense Mozart's joy in composing this, or as if to say: "So the Parisians are sophisticates? Let this melt them down to size!"

It takes no rocket scientist to tell us why this captivates us. We are rhythmic and harmonic creatures existing always within the potentially disruptive onslaught of the much-at-once. Mozart's symphony attunes us, tunes us up, saves us from the threat of chaos or madness, panic or boredom. Perhaps, in ultimate humming and delighted life, this music resonates with three beats of the heart to one inhale and expiration of the lungs; perhaps this metarhythm is optimal normative, for the human organism—and possibly also for some nonhuman sorts. Nothing is more powerfully impelling and moving than is our own well functioning as organism-selves. The term Aristotle uses is *eudaimonia*, inadequately translated into English as "happiness," which indicates all the capacities of the soul reaching their excellence through an attunement with the particularities of the situation in which the organism finds itself. Perhaps the best we can do in English is "well functioning," though I prefer "humming."

Likewise, the brain oscillates rhythmically in many ways. For example, Evan Thompson writes, "According to a neurodynamical perspective, mental states are embodied in large-scale dynamical patterns of brain activity . . . and these patterns both emerge from distributed, local activities and also globally shape or constrain these local activities. One can thus conjecture that . . . large-scale brain activity shifts from one coherent global pattern to another, and thereby entrains local neural processes" ("Neurophenomenology and Contemplative Experience," 231). In shifting from one global pattern to another, and thereby entraining local neural processes, music can free us—at least for the moment—from fixations and hang-ups to development, and sensitize us to the movements and rhythms of the environing much-at-once. Music, as well as contemplative experience, can free us to realize our inherent potential as organism-selves to ripen reliably and regeneratively into mature life. It can unleash that immensely powerful urge to "become what we are," or who we are, as thinkers from Aristotle to Nietzsche have pointed out.

It might seem that we need only look into our brains with ever-more-sophisticated and discriminating brain-scan instruments to find out the "neuronal basis" of our lives, or "who we really are." But whoa! We have been supposing all along that it is bodily *selves* who develop powerfully toward maturation, but the concept or word *self* cannot figure in the reports that brain scientists qua brain scientists deliver to us. They must limit themselves to the glossary of terms useable by science: that is, to factual reports in physiological and biological terms of complex neural networks, say, or of microvolts across synapses of neurons, or of oscillations of networks in certain mathematically determinable frequencies.

Nor is this merely a "scholastic," "academic," or "verbal" point. Evolution has seen to it, apparently, that we can have no direct awareness of our own brains. As mentioned above, if we had had this capacity, then probably our awareness would have been so cluttered that our ability to react quickly enough to survive in emergencies would have been seriously compromised. In one sense, our awareness *is* simply our lives lived immediately within our own complex neural, glandular, and skeletal organisms. But we can only know what our awareness *is* in the much fuller sense when we know what our awareness is *of* or *about* in the context of the world that holds us. As Dewey put it schematically, the actual operant unit is not "mind" or "brain" alone—or "body" alone—but brain-in-body-in-environment. Hegel put this synoptically and succinctly in his own way: The earth is not the physical center of the universe, but is the metaphysical center. That is, only in the "hawk's-eye view" of the whole earth, and our place and funded behavior within it, can the *meaning* of all things be discovered to reside. The so-called mind/body problem is not that of connecting separate substances or entities—mental and physical—but is that of connecting different regions or levels of conceptualization and discourse. Even the meaning of "volt"—as in "microvolt"—has been established within the earth of funded human interactions. In this case, the name is in honor of Italian physicist Alessandro Volta (1745–1827), who first formulated that unit of electrical reality.

We are on the scent of why brain science and the "simple art of observation" must work in tandem, as Oliver Sacks has asserted. Sacks supplies an example of the great need to do this; he relates how he and a colleague disputed whether a patient suffering from severe Alzheimer's disease had lost his *self* (*Musicophilia,* 335ff.). He resisted agreeing that the patient had lost his self, but finally wondered if he and his colleague were really disagreeing. It was easily conceivable that Sacks and his colleague agreed on all the available brain facts but kept disagreeing about the status of the self; if so, they were disagreeing about how the self should be conceptualized. (I hope that Sacks did not conclude that he and his colleague were not really disagreeing, because that would be to assume that one can really disagree only about "empirical facts," not about material essences and meanings, such as the meaning of *self.* That would be an insidious form of reductionism—in fact, a form of nihilism.)

Even if a person, say, Caleb Robinson, lies dead in his coffin, we may hesitate an instant before saying that this is no longer he, his *self*—though radically altered—a dead body that once was Caleb. How the self may or may not mesh with the world and its rhythms even after death remains a mystery. So dense is the world in which we must try to find our way! So easy is it for us to jump to conclusions—to be jumpy and fearful—to mangle and reduce the meaning and *being* of our lives.

Here, with regard to the conceptualization of essences, the chief twentieth-century phenomenologist Edmund Husserl gave us an important clue. He wrote of essences of things as the sets of features that things must possess if they are to count as *being* those things—thus "essential" features. In other words, we cannot *mean* them or refer to them without assuming that they possess these features. Husserl characterized formal essences—such as "triangle"—as those with fixed, clear scopes of application. Given the accepted definition of triangle, figures are either such or they are not. Husserl then characterized "material essences" or, provocatively, "experimental essences" as those with floating scopes of application. In some key cases, we may not agree whether they apply. But this vagueness is not necessarily a defect, as Charles Peirce pointed out vehemently, for the actual world in which we live and must make or find meaning—the much-at-once—is endlessly dense, "rich" in Sacks's language, indeed, bottomless in its meaning-potential for our experience. It could be that the "vague" is all we have! It could be that living, vital "essences" are themselves in their outlines and transformations vague!

Another case presented by Sacks challenges our powers of conceptualization even more. He writes of a man profoundly afflicted with Parkinson's disease who most of the time doesn't look like the same person as he formerly appeared. When he is caught up in music, however, it is as though his old self reemerges.

> It is music that the Parkinsonian needs, for only music, which is rigorous yet spacious, sinuous and alive, can evoke responses that are equally so. And he needs not only the metrical structure of rhythm and the free movement of melody—its contours and trajectories, its ups and downs, its tensions and relaxations—but the "will" and intentionality of music, to allow him to regain the freedom of his own kinetic melody. (*Musicophilia*, 258)

Can we say that the old self reemerges? Do we imply that it was hidden somewhere previously? Where and in what form exactly? Isn't it more accurate to say that it is reconstituted? For it is deceptive to assume that the self is a strange substance that must remain itself through time—even as it loses some "accidental" attributes for a while—as long as it exists at all. But if we give up continuity as an essential feature, we are at a loss to say just what its essential attributes are. What are we to make of Sacks's intriguing allusion to one's "own kinetic melody"? Can't one pick up one's rhythm and melody again, without it being an underlying substance, but being instead more of a joint performance undertaken again with the world's rhythms?

This is strange, vague, perplexing. I surmise that we humans are inherently paradoxical and unstable creatures, and I do not know how unstable we can be and still be ourselves. The concept of self floats *exceedingly*. But if that's a truth about us, what could be more importantly true than a truth of our own selves? It will guide our conduct. We will be very cautious about giving up on human selves, whether our own or another's. Besides, can't we imagine that being perplexed about something is, in some cases, an indication that we are in touch with something truly fundamental? But just which cases? We don't dare block the road of inquiry.

My way of trying to reduce the dangers of jumping to conclusions and of reductionism in this book has been to open up the meaning of sound and music in our lives. An ever-increasing number of thinkers avoid reductionism by being phenomenological in key ways. A remarkable effort is Shaun Gallagher's 1997 article "Mutual Enlightenment: Recent Phenomenology in Cognitive Science" and his 2005 book *How the Body Shapes the Mind*. With remarkable patience, nimbleness, and a many-sidedness of approach, he keeps open possibilities for discovering meaning, refusing to jump to conclusions, keeping open the road of inquiry, as Peirce would say, over the long term. The commodiousness, the room to maneuver, the fresh air is palpable, regenerating, and refreshing. Gallagher sees that close attention to our "mental life" may lead to fruitful hypotheses about "brain states," and that, contrariwise, our attention to the latter afforded by ever-improving brain-scanning instruments may prompt us to look into previously overlooked corners and crevices of our lives as we live them immediately.

To understand *why* brain science and what Sacks calls the "simple art of observation" must work together has become more difficult in our secularized culture than we typically imagine. It used to be, say, that a concept of *self* was secured by linking it to *soul*, the latter construed as created by God and as immaterial, outliving the body; meanwhile, world and cosmos were likewise secured as created by God. Now our basic concepts have a way of hanging in the air, flitting about, eluding our firm grasp. Only Nietzsche, I think, grasps anything like the full consequences of his fictional madman's cry, "God is dead!" (*The Gay Science,* §125). Nietzsche creates a brilliant metaphor, building on the scientific fact that in the late nineteenth century the speed of light had been measured—a metaphor that is endlessly suggestive. Belief in God, he writes, is like a distant star that has burned out: its light still reaches us, but the source of the star's light and heat—this immense roiling cauldron of energy—is extinguished.

The danger is to think that *self* is only a word—an objectionably vague one at that—or that these issues with which we struggle are merely arcane or academic. We are trying to get purchase on the most concrete and momentous matters, yet also the most slippery. To wit, a firm in my own town claims to treat and cure addiction with the advertisement:

> Our Revolutionary and Unique Medical Treatments focus on the Neurochemical imbalances in the brain. These imbalances Cause the Uncontrollable Cravings that lead to Drug and Alcohol Addiction.

This is a serious oversimplification. What is true is that certain brain states are the necessary condition for addictive cravings, so that if these are eliminated the cravings cease—at least for a time. This is not unimportant, as their elimination may prevent suicide, for example, and may "buy time" to rediscover one's attunement as brain-in-body-in-environment.

But to assert they are the "cause" is to block recognition of a whole manner of living in the world that is probably not self-compounding, not regenerative, not importantly creative or free. It is to mask out a failure of *meaning* in one's self and life, and also to mask out the masking out. Can we say that the chief challenge today is to retrieve and reinterpret what self as *soul* could possibly be?

From the beginning of this book I have tried to avoid that rigid gazing and fixing on things that is so typical of vision—that takes "I see" as equivalent to "I understand." Nor is it sufficient to emphasize the freedom, capaciousness, and spontaneity of *glancing* over fixed *gazing* and its twin, *measuring*. I have countered that tendency to fix on the secular, leaving it segregated from the sacred, for in our actual living, things that are isolated by the abstractions of verbal intellect flow together, particularly in intense moments of our participation; they merge and meld into each other. Thus I have tried to affirm William James's critique of "vicious intellectualism." I want to be active, balanced, poised, able to jump nimbly from one level of meaning to another, keeping insights and perspectives assembled, whole. Hence, among other things, I have honored the powers of metaphor.

What happens when we emphasize hearing, sound, music, and say that knowing is at least as much *like that* as is seeing-gazing? What if the auditory becomes *proton analagon*? We are better prepared to expect something that comes from any direction at any time, when we are "just playing" or dreaming—musing as Peirce put it—or when, in Emerson's words, "pre-cantations, which sail like odors in the air" ("The Poet," in *Nature and Selected Essays*, 273) arise, hypotheses in germinal form that might break through encrusted habit and trance. Finally we will discern how, for example, the meaning of *soul* bleeds into *self*. We will not be satisfied with reductionist accounts of meaning, no matter how "authoritative," intricate, or clever.

There is an apparently anomalous volume in the Library of Living Philosophers entitled *Albert Einstein, Philosopher-Scientist*, which is apt here because Einstein's genius and character add weight to the power of sound, music, play, spontaneity. His autobiographical note in the volume records his intense rejection of coercion, both obvious and subtle, in modern education. This includes the coercion exacted by preoccupation with frequent examinations—for this requires us to focus on what *others*, counted as authorities, believe to be of importance. These authorities may be at bottom conventional souls, afraid of leaps of imagination, not open to the insights that come only to those who tingle in their deepest roots in response to the much-at-once: that fertile darkness that comes only to individual points within itself at particular moments.

> It is . . . nothing short of a miracle that the modern methods of instruction have not yet entirely strangled the holy [*heilige*] curiosity of inquiry; for this delicate little plant, aside from stimulation, stands mainly in need of freedom; without this it goes to wreck and ruin without fail. It is a very grave mistake to think that the enjoyment of seeing and searching can be promoted by means of coercion and a sense of duty. To the contrary, I believe that it would be possible to rob even a healthy beast of prey of its voraciousness, if it were possible, with the aid of a whip, to force the beast to devour continuously, even when not hungry. (*Albert Einstein, Philosopher-Scientist,* 17)

Not the least of the power of this passage is Einstein's allusion to beasts of prey and to ill-fated attempts to overwhelm their instinctive cycles and rhythms of appetite with whips. We have our own appetites, including those of *comprehending* the world. We learn best when we hunger to do so and act on our hunger whenever we feel it. Learning and knowing come from the joyful periodic exercise of animal energy.

APPENDIX C

THE BODY-SCHEMA AND DIMENSIONS OF EMPATHY

Recent experiments with technologically generated perceptual illusion resonate well with the argument of this book because they suggest that primal empathy between selves is not committed in advance to psychophysical dualisms or self/other binary oppositions. In the study by Valeria I. Petkova and H. Henrik Ehrsson, "If I Were You: Perceptual Illusion of Body Swapping" (summarized in *New York Times*, December 2, 2008), an experimenter and a subject sit on chairs facing each other. The experimenter is equipped with electronic goggles that broadcast images of his own hands and arms, as they appear presently deployed to himself, to the subject's goggles. The first-person reality of the experimenter's hands and arms thus appear in the field and on the margins of the subject's goggled vision, giving way to his unseen trunk. When this sight appears in the subject's goggles, the subject realizes that these hands and arms are not his own, and is startled—perhaps disturbed—by the sight of them.

The reasons for being startled and even disturbed are not far to seek. For throughout one's life, only one's own body has appeared from this unique first-person viewpoint. When one's hands and arms lie in one's lap, only they and one's lap appear, the remainder of one's body does not.

It is that singular body that is ever close and warm and, as James put it, "the storm center of all this stress" through time: that is, the history, indeed the being, of one's self (see James's crucial footnote in "The Experience of Activity," 211n1). For that surely is the implication James wishes us to draw: that the self is not some unverifiable nonextended mental substance somehow hidden away inside one and open immediately only to its own mental "contents," such as, for example, "afterimages." Rather, the self essentially involves one's active body and, when we are aware, our unique experiencing of it through time. How else to explain why persons mentally and emotionally ill-balanced tend to be more than startled, even badly disturbed, by the experience mediated by the goggles, according to the study. For the underpinnings of their very selves are threatened. They experience ontological anxiety or panic.

This electronic technology, it seems, has obscured something fundamental without throwing it completely out of action. To understand how the technology can be both revealing and disruptive of normal functioning, we must understand the latter (and I'm not sure that the experimenters adequately do). If one—ungoggled—attempts to reflect on one's own prereflective, effective, ongoing bodily activity as it is actually happening here and now—either the everyday sort or as an artist or athlete—one badly fouls it up. It no longer uncoils as one's self in action, flowing like a silken ribbon from a frictionless spool, for one is "self-conscious" in the pitiable, self-destructive sense.

Differently put, we best speak of the normally and typically experienced body-schema, not the body image, which implies something static (see Shaun Gallagher, *How the Body Shapes the Mind*)—a fundamental distinction not made, apparently, by the experimenters. That is, the body-schema invokes the normal and habitual adaptive routes through the world-as-experienced taken by one's body-self, some of which involve awareness, but the primal sort being prereflective. These inherently first-person activities are self-evidently *mine,* and as they continue as wholly *mine* they constitute the primordial reality of self. This anchoring of mineness or selfhood in the body-schema holds even when particular actions are spontaneous, done for the first time. Body-schemas cannot be reduced to "mental contents," such as sensory images or afterimages in an essentially reflective "mind."

Of course, we emphatically do not live in isolation, and properly interpreted, the experiments can help us understand empathy. Without basal empathy with a range of others we couldn't *be* at all. We must have primal empathy because without it we couldn't mimetically absorb the set of distinctive body-schemas of other persons in our culture that form our experienced and experienceable world, and there is evidence that correlatively this basal empathy with others "embeds" their capacities in our own body schema. That is, without it, human organisms couldn't be conditioned generation after generation to coordinate the foci of their attention, to notice what others in their group notice, fail to notice what others fail to do, and so on. That is, without it there couldn't emerge that shared cultural reality—the culture's experienced and experienceable world—which all must share if each is to be accounted normal and sane.

The experiments in question do reveal just how primal this empathy must be: They show how empathy can even be forced, as it were, in some circumstances. For example, if the experimenter is African and the subject Caucasian, there is some evidence that this goggled experience diminishes the subject's racial prejudice, if it has previously existed, according to the *New York Times* article. Thus we might better discern why segregation—separation of the races—was so vehemently demanded by slave states—because primal empathy tends to be contagious. But perhaps this odd experience of primal empathy is just an artifact of this ingenious electronic technology, and not true in any way of the actual life that we live everyday? There is good reason to think that the technology—"larger than life"—has alerted us to something that does indeed go on in everyday life, but is typically overlooked. If so, it is perhaps overlooked because of embedded dualistic Cartesian assumptions concerning private, personal, mental substance, with their "contents," buried from others but somehow inside each of us, directly and immediately intuitable and reportable by each.

The experimenters proceeded to do more work on empathy by employing a human-form mannequin as seen from its own "point of view," with this first-person point of view broadcast again directly into the subject's goggles. Though what is seen is clearly a mannequin, not an actual human person, identification and deep empathy with the mannequin—in this case—again appears. This experiment bears out yet again that awareness here is *sciousness,* as James calls it—prereflective and prevoluntary—not consciousness, or awareness of awareness, which involves one's powerful body-schema and the primal awareness that goes along with it.

An interesting wrinkle shows up here. In order for the illusion to hold that one is empathizing with a *human being,* the subject's actual body must be stimulated. This is particularly true if the mannequin's abdomen, say, is "threatened" with a knife, with this seen, of course, in the subject's goggles from the mannequin's "point of view." For the illusion to hold, the subject's abdomen is stimulated out of his sight with a short rod, either synchronously or asynchronously with the threatened knife-puncture of the mannequin's abdomen. The eyes, of course, play a fundamental role, but as we might anticipate, are not all-important. In order to demonstrate that the subject is really identifying with the mannequin, the experimenters employ skin conductivity tests (they declare their desire for "objective truth" about the illusion and what makes it possible, as they want to establish their credentials as *scientists*—and here they reveal something of what they mean by science).

In general, if we know just what it is that obscures or derails normal perception and creates an illusion, we will better know what makes normal perception possible. We who interpret the experimenters' experiments can see that it is the body-schema of the active body-self that is temporarily derailed—or at least temporarily obscured—and we better learn its normally great powers and properties. These experiments, when liberally and knowledgeably construed, expand our understanding of mirror neurons (discussed in Segment 4, note 2), because we better place them in the actual context of the active everyday life of brain-in-body-in-environment. This all suggests, of course, that one's identity as a self is far more tied to the body interacting with the environment than the private, Cartesian, nonextended mental-substance theory would or could anticipate.

If we ask why seeing a part of a body is seeing the whole body—the whole body-self—the answer is not far to seek. For the body-schema normally animates the entire effectively functioning body-self. Parts are directly experienced as parts-of-wholes. Organs are experienced as members of an ensemble that functions for the sake of the whole. So then, to see the part is to see the whole. Eyes are organs attached to the skull by muscles and nerves, and indeed when things are functioning right, the skull is that of a whole body stanced to engage effectively with the world. Eyes, hands, the whole body act for the sake of the whole-body-in-the-world. The normal reality is surpassingly organismic, and when things are humming along, the reality is self-compounding, self-rectifying, and self-equilibrating—it is fugal.

Here it should be clear that I am elaborating on the experimenters' work, for the experimenters seem not to adequately grasp this organismic reality and our experience of it. They find it "remarkable" that when the subject equipped with the goggles shakes hands with the experimenter, the subject feels the pressure in the *other*'s hand. But we must remember that an image of that other's hand has been overlaid on the subject's body-schema, and that—even though overshadowed by the technology—in the end the body-schema trumps the image without entirely displacing it. Though in the moment the experience may be remarkable, even weird, it is not remarkable or weird in the sense of being inexplicable. It is explained in the context of the full organismic reality of the normal situation that our own body schema is not isolated but envelops others.

It is *listening*, along with the whole array of auditory metaphors, that can reveal this possibility of deep, normal, ongoing, prevoluntary and predeliberate empathy with others, human or not, by snatching it out of the glare of seeing and the visual metaphors that usually eclipse it. For, when we are animated and dilated, even relaxed by the auditory, we no longer fixedly gaze at and objectify other's bodies "out there"—in the third-person point of view—but allow their bodies as immediately perceived and felt by them to move fully and fluidly *through us* in the much-at-once, just as these bodily others are living their lives in the first-person. That is for them to take possession of us to one degree or another. We certainly don't squint at these strange creatures surrounding us in puzzlement, but interlock with them in the experience, as when we hear music together and our bodies sway in time and rhythm as a corporate body! Sometimes we are so entranced as to be de facto hypnotized by them, deeply enthralled. Noticing persons attending a Hitler-style rally—or adoring young fans at a big rock concert—should make this obvious. Consider also how we can immediately empathize with animals.

To detect the actual interfusions, the primal empathy that is occurring in *sciousness* without the aid of electronic technology is immensely difficult for many of us. This is because the sclerotic conceptual distinctions and polarizations that structure and greatly affect our "mysterious sensorial life" (James) of body/mind and self/other are so deeply and habitually engrained. That the other's *first-person* experiencing very often bleeds into one's own—how can this be? But it happens! If we look attentively and calmly for it, there is considerable evidence for that. Recall, for example, that mirror neurons were discovered practically by accident. While a baboon's brain activity was lighting up the brain-scan screen in the lab, it saw an assistant eating an ice cream cone, and the scan was then recording what it would have if the baboon itself had been eating. Happily, this fact was noticed at the time, not immediately passed over and suppressed as "impossible."

If others are experienced, by contrast, as profoundly alien or dangerous, we may feel violated, polluted, revolted by them (see Wilshire, *Get 'Em All! Kill 'Em!: Genocide, Terrorism, Righteous Communities*). Ironically, only our porousness and vulnerability, incident upon our tendency to deeply empathize, can explain how this happens. For only when this profound tendency to empathize is overridden by deep fear, confusion, or revulsion can we seek violently to extrude those others from their entrenchment *within us*. Then genocide appears as a live and tempting possibility.

The very art and livelihood of excellent actors depends on their ability to tap this form of possession or deep empathy. After Marlon Brando's death, one of his friends cited an incident from his life: while watching a train of migrating ants, Brando is quoted as saying, "Do you think if we watched them long enough, we could walk as they do?" Perhaps one reason Brando notoriously undervalued both stage and screen theater was that deep empathy and deep enactment came so easily to him? Of course, the Strasberg Method of taking on the affective sense of the world of characters by also taking on the sense of their bodies and perceptual reality had undoubtedly strengthened those capacities Brando possessed originally.

The intellectualist tradition of equating mind with consciousness—with the activity of a private mental substance open immediately only to its own reflective inventorying and verbal report of its "contents"—has badly impeded our understanding of ourselves as a species. As Darwin tersely noted, "Origin of man now proved—he who understands baboon would do more towards metaphysics than Locke" (*Notebook M*, 1838, quoted in Cheney and Seyfarth, *Baboon Metaphysics: The Evolution of a Social Mind*, 1). Under the influence of Descartes's idea of mind as private reflective consciousness, John Locke equated the identity of a human qua person with the continuity of his or her memories back through time, cumulatively identified by him or her as *mine*. But because one has no memory of being born, this leads to the absurdity that as a person one "has no mother"; by this I mean that the sense of having been brought into this world, birthed and nurtured by kin, is a felt bodily sense of the deep past, yet is nowhere to be found in our recollections or "mental memories." If we didn't have this bodily hold on the deep past, before any reflective memories, we wouldn't have the feeling of belonging to the earth and to our kin. The experiments prompt us to revisit the whole question of self and its multiplex aspects: crevices, alveoli, interfusions, echoes. As bodily beings, we are intercorporeal, open on all sides every moment to others and to other things, actual and possible. We are beings that can act voluntarily and take responsibility for acting morally and companionably—which we easily fail to do.

Only when we consider ourselves in our true organismic wholeness can we begin to grasp the profound perplexities and agonies of addiction, to broach a prime example. As I elaborated in *Wild Hunger: The Primal Roots of Modern Addiction*, addiction is an agonizingly *confusing* experience—often to the point of totally incapacitating us for remedial action. Because a craving is experienced ineluctably as the work and process of my own body, it is definitely primordially *mine*, the work of *my self*. But because my sense of self also includes, ineluctably, my sense of ability to control myself, unforced by the "external" world, when I cannot control the craving it is simultaneously experienced as *not mine*. *Mine* and *not mine* at once—leading to diabolical confusion and disturbing dissonance. In other words, we are always "beyond ourselves" in the sense of our isolated selves, whereas in our primal embodiment, even in pathological states, we never lose the sense of being enveloped in the much-at-once.

Our difficulties in understanding ourselves are far indeed from being merely theoretical. Affected are our abilities, for instance, to evaluate candidates for the highest offices of the land. We have a prime example in Ronald Reagan (see William F. Buckley Jr., *The Reagan I Knew*). People were astonished at how little they could learn about his "interior" or "personal" life: that is, his thoughts and aspirations, likes and dislikes, feelings, and so on. One interviewer used this metaphor: Asking him a personal question was like dropping a stone in a well and then hearing no sound at all.

Yet Reagan was a powerfully minding person and organism in a very significant sense. In Nietzsche's phrase, he would "shoot out a shining star" and be pulled irresistibly toward it. Reagan can be said to have deeply identified with—to have empathized with—the shining star. He was strongly purposive and end-directed; "the star" claimed his consuming interest and devotion (recall that double emphasis in the preface and prologue). As a young lifeguard in the Midwest he saved the lives of dozens of people. One might empathically imagine him swimming in a tunnel of his own bubbles toward the desperate victim. As president of the Screen Actors Guild, his life and the lives of his family were threatened by communist labor organizers and he was licensed to carry a pistol. The "private man" in his deliberate conduct was continually reaching beyond himself in acts of taking in others! Clearly, as president of the United States, once he fixed his minding on eliminating the "evil empire," the USSR, there was no stopping him, the burden was his as the "shining star." How are we to evaluate Reagan's "mind" and "self"? First of all, we have to be as sure as we can that we have expanded and deepened what we mean by these terms. They must mean more than introspective loquacity or self-centered talkativeness. Would he have been a better president if he had been more obviously reflective?

I think these questions are not resolvable because a mystery about the human condition must remain, stemming from our insertion in a deep past of primal life and the history of the planet, as well as our bodily incorporation in the teeming life of the planet, in myriad others, some human, some more-than-human. I am suggesting, however, that it is not the reflective capacities of Reagan, or anyone else for that matter, that is the key to understanding their life trajectory and talents, but rather their way of being part of a deeper musical sense of the world that our literal musical creations express but can never fully fathom or exhaust.

AFTERWORD

Gil Wilshire

I have powerful memories of my father surrounding himself with music. The house was always filled with classical music played at nine-tenths volume. All the great composers were featured, although Bruckner—what he called "Big Music"—was perhaps his favorite. Music was the wellspring of rejuvenation in which my father found solace and deep understanding. It is fitting that Bruce's last major philosophical work engages this subject.

This final book fittingly outlines the fugue that was my father's life. In his late teens, recurrent pneumonia kept him stateside during the Korean War. An Army desk assignment in Atlanta exposed him to acting, a profession alien to his upbringing. He was handsome, with a booming voice, and began landing roles in the theater. An Army drill sergeant commented in his southern drawl, "Will-Shire, where do you get them wurds?" Bruce's vocabulary was already prodigious. Moving to New York City, he met my mother, Donna, an aspiring actress. Their long marriage and collaboration shaped all his works. His *Role Playing and Identity* (1982) derives from the unique insights gained in his thespian pursuits and international performance studies. His PhD dissertation was on the work of William James—often considered foremost a psychologist—whose influence pervaded Bruce's thoughts. My father also had chronic pain from a badly damaged knee and back problems. He again turned lemons into lemonade by working with his infirmities through the techniques of F. M. Alexander and Moshe Feldenkrais. These insights, developed in his essays on healing, penetrate many of his other works. Perhaps the most poignant intellectual sublimation of his life was the reaction he and his family had to the sudden death of his cherished daughter, Rebekah, at age thirty-one after a horseback riding accident. Out of the emotional ashes came his book *Get 'Em all! Kill 'Em!* (2004). He stated that only by studying a subject more horrible than the death of a child could he eke out a modicum of solace and probity. As the dirge section of his fugue continued in the aftermath of Rebekah's death, the maladaptive behavior of an addiction struck his family. He was never one to lose insight from these teachable moments, and his book *Wild Hunger* (1998) was born. The musical strains of Bruce's life did grow joyous and fulfilling once again. In the present final work, composed in the years around retirement, the various strands and ideas of his career are interwoven and all the chords and dissonances are resolved.

He was just entering retirement and preparing to put the final touches on this manuscript when he suffered an aortic dissection: a sudden vascular catastrophe that kills the large majority of its sufferers. My father's heart was strong from his years in the mountains, and he survived, but the event took its toll and he was not able to see the completed manuscript into print. His loving wife of more than fifty years, Donna, made polishing revisions over the following year. The two were a lifelong team and their numerous works always involved collaboration; she would read her modifications to him, and he approved them after consensual feedback.

When cancer suddenly took Donna's life, the ensuing events made progress toward publication challenging. At this time two of Bruce's dearest colleague-friends, Glen A. Mazis and Edward S. Casey, took it upon themselves to guide the project to publication. Bruce loved both these men for their friendship, loyalty, and collegial support over many years. I am deeply grateful for their contribution.

The manuscript has also benefited greatly from the professional developmental editing of Lissa McCullough, a notably talented and experienced person in the field. She brought the manuscript into final publishable form.

Bruce finally succumbed to this series of adversities on January 1, 2013, surrounded by family and friends. He lived a good life. His ashes lie with those of his wife, Donna, and daughter, Rebekah, at high altitude in the magnificent beauty of the Sierra Mountains. I feel blessed to have ever-present memories of him to guide me and to pass on to the next generation. I hope this book enhances its readers' understanding of life in some of the ways my father's philosophical insights have enriched mine. For those wishing to feel Bruce's presence, hear his great voice, experience his natural humor, and witness his knowledge of history, there is a delightful twenty-minute video of him discussing his coin collection on YouTube: https://www.youtube.com/watch?v=456_J70P1a4.

Works Cited

Abram, David. *Becoming Animal: An Earthly Cosmology.* New York: Random House, 2010.

———. *The Spell of the Sensuous: Perception and Language in a More-than-Human World.* New York: Pantheon, 1996.

Ackerman, Diane. *An Alchemy of Mind: The Marvel and Mystery of the Brain.* New York: Scribner, 2004.

Arendt, Hannah. *Eichmann in Jerusalem: A Report on the Banality of Evil.* New York: Penguin, 1994.

Barrett, William. *The Illusion of Technique: A Search for Meaning in a Technological Civilization.* Garden City, N.Y.: Doubleday-Anchor, 1978.

———. *Irrational Man: A Study in Existential Philosophy.* Garden City, N.Y.: Doubleday-Anchor, 1958.

———. *Time of Need: Forms of Imagination in the Twentieth Century.* New York: Harper & Row, 1972.

Beasley, Conger, Jr. "In Animals We Find Ourselves." *Orion: Nature Quarterly* 9, no.2 (spring 1990): 16–23.

Beckett, Samuel. *Waiting for Godot: A Tragicomedy in Two Acts.* New York: Grove, 1954.

Bellow, Saul. *The Adventures of Augie March.* Fiftieth Anniversary Edition. Introduction by Christopher Hitchens. New York: Penguin, 2003.

Berry, Thomas. *The Dream of the Earth.* San Francisco: Sierra Club Books, 1988.

Blake, William. *The Marriage of Heaven and Hell.* In *The Complete Poetry and Prose of William Blake.* Newly Revised Edition. Edited by David V. Erdman. Commentary by Harold Bloom. Berkeley: University of California Press, 1982.

Bloom, Harold. *The American Religion: The Emergence of the Post-Christian Nation.* New York: Simon & Schuster, 1992.

Bohm, David. *Wholeness and the Implicate Order.* London: Routledge and Kegan Paul, 1980.

Boito, Arrigo. *Nerone.* Hungarian State Opera. Eve Queler. Hungaroton HCD12487-89, 3 compact discs

———. *Nerone*. RAI Torino. Gianandrea Gavazzeni. Living Stage 2110539, 2 compact discs.

Bradshaw, Gay. *Elephants on the Edge: What Animals Teach Us about Humanity*. New Haven: Yale University Press, 2009.

The Bridge. Documentary film directed and produced by Eric Steel. DVD. Koch Lorger Films, 2008.

Brook, Peter. "About *Tierno Bokar*." Program Notes, November 19, 2004. http://www.tiernobokar.columbia.edu/pdfs/brook_bocar.pdf

Bruckner, Anton. Symphony no. 9 (with Documentation of the Finale Fragment). Vienna Philharmonic Orchestra. Nikolaus Harnoncourt. RCA SACD 54332, 2 compact discs.

Buber, Martin. *Between Man and Man*. 1947. New York: Macmillan, 1965.

Buckley, William F., Jr. *The Reagan I Knew*. New York: Basic, 2008.

Bugbee, Henry. *The Inward Morning: A Philosophical Exploration in Journal Form*. 1958. Introduction by Edward F. Mooney. Athens, Ga.: University of Georgia Press, 1999.

Casey, Edward S. *The World at a Glance*. Bloomington: Indiana University Press, 2007.

Chambers, Oswald. *Devotions for Morning and Evening with Oswald Chambers: My Utmost for His Highest*. Cleveland, Oh.: World Publishing, 2002.

Cheney, Dorothy L., and Robert M. Seyfarth. *Baboon Metaphysics: The Evolution of a Social Mind*. Chicago: University of Chicago Press, 2007.

Chernow, Ron. *Alexander Hamilton*. New York: Penguin, 2004.

Chorost, Michael. *Rebuilt: My Journey Back to the Hearing World*. New York: Houghton Mifflin Harcourt, 2005.

Clark, Ronald W. *Einstein: The Life and Times. An Illustrated Biography*. New York: Abrams, 1984.

Damasio, Antonio R. *Descartes' Error: Emotion, Reason, and the Human Brain*. New York: Putnam's Sons, 1994.

Dewey, John. *Art as Experience*. 1934. New York: Capricorn, 2005.

———. *Experience and Nature*. 1929. 2nd ed. New York: Dover, 1958.

———. *Logic: The Theory of Inquiry*. 1938. New York: Holt, Rinehart, and Winston, 1964.

Dodds, E. R. *The Greeks and the Irrational*. Berkeley: University of California Press, 1951.

Ehrenreich, Barbara. *Dancing in the Streets: A History of Collective Joy*. New York: Metropolitan, 2007.

Einstein, Albert. *Albert Einstein, Philosopher-Scientist*. Edited by Paul Arthur Schilpp. Library of Living Philosophers, vol. 7. 3rd ed. Chicago: Open Court, 1998.

Einstein, Alfred. *Mozart: His Character, His Work.* Oxford: Oxford University Press, 1965.

Emerson, Ralph Waldo. *Nature and Selected Essays.* Edited by Larzer Ziff. New York: Penguin, 1982.

———. "Poetry and Imagination." In *The Works of Ralph Waldo Emerson.* Fireside Edition. 12 vols. Boston, 1909.

Emoto, Masuru. *The True Power of Water: Healing and Discovering Ourselves.* New York: Atria, 2005.

Faulkner, William. Nobel Prize address. In *The Faulkner Reader.* New York: Random House, 1954.

Feldenkrais, Moshe. *Body and Mature Behavior: A Study of Anxiety, Sex, Gravitation and Learning.* 1949. New York: International Universities Press, 1979.

Foote, Shelby. *The Civil War: A Narrative.* 3 vols. New York: Random House, 1958–74.

Gallagher, Shaun. *How the Body Shapes the Mind.* Oxford: Oxford University Press, 2005.

———. "Mutual Enlightenment: Recent Phenomenology in Cognitive Science." *Journal of Consciousness Studies* 4, no. 3 (1997): 195–214.

Gebser, Jean. *The Ever-Present Origin.* Translated by Noel Barstad and Algis Mickunas. Athens: Ohio University Press, 1986.

Gendlin, Eugene. "Introduction to 'Thinking at the Edge.'" *The Folio: A Journal for Focusing and Experimental Therapy* 19, no. 1 (2004): 1–8.

Gerber, Richard. *Vibrational Medicine: The #1 Handbook of Subtle-Energy Therapies.* Rochester, Vt.: Bear and Company, 2001.

Gibbon, Edward. *Decline and Fall of the Roman Empire.* Hertfordshire, England: Wordsworth Editions, 1998.

Glass, Philip, and Robert Wilson. *Einstein on the Beach.* The Philip Glass Ensemble. Michael Riesman. Recorded 1996. Nonesuch B000005J28, 2012, 3 compact discs.

Glover, Danny. Speech at Higher Ground Hurricane Relief Benefit jazz concert, Lincoln Center, September 17, 2005. Republished in "Belafonte & Glover Speak Out on Katrina." Alternet, September 22, 2005. http://www.alternet.org/story/25862/belafonte_%26_glover_speak_out_on_katrina

Goodman, Felicitas D. *Ecstasy, Ritual, and Alternate Reality: Religion in a Pluralistic World.* Bloomington: Indiana University Press, 1988.

———. *Where the Spirits Ride the Wind: Trance Journeys and Other Ecstatic Experiences.* Bloomington: Indiana University Press, 1990.

Hadamard, Jacques. *The Mathematician's Mind: The Psychology of Invention in the Mathematical Field.* With a new preface by P. N. Johnson-Laird. Princeton: Princeton University Press, 1996.

Halton, Eugene. *Bereft of Reason: On the Decline of Social Thought and Prospects for Its Renewal.* Chicago: University of Chicago Press, 1995.

———. *Meaning and Modernity: Social Theory in the Pragmatic Attitude.* Chicago: University of Chicago Press, 1986.

———. "Peircian Animism and the End of Civilization," *Contemporary Pragmatism* 2, no. 1 (June 2005): 135–66.

Heidegger, Martin. *Off the Beaten Track.* Translated by Julian Young and Kenneth Haynes. Cambridge: Cambridge University Press, 2002.

Hofstadter, Douglas. *I Am a Strange Loop.* New York: Basic Books, 2007.

Hölderlin, Friedrich. "Patmos." In *Hyperion and Selected Poems*, 244–55. New York: Continuum, 1990.

James, William. "The Experience of Activity," "On a Certain Blindness in Human Beings," "The Perception of Reality," and "The Place of Affectional Facts in a World of Pure Experience." In *William James: The Essential Writings.* Edited by Bruce W. Wilshire. Preface by James M. Edie. New York: Harper & Row, 1971.

———. "Is Life Worth Living?" in *The Will to Believe and Other Essays in Popular Philosophy*, 32–62. New York: Dover, 1956:

———. *The Principles of Psychology.* 1890. 3 vols. Cambridge, Mass.: Harvard University Press, 1981.

———. *Some Problems of Philosophy.* Introduction by Peter H. Hare. Foreword by Frederick H. Burkhardt. Cambridge, Mass.: Harvard University Press, 1979.

———. *The Varieties of Religious Experience.* Introduction by John E. Smith. Cambridge, Mass.: Harvard University Press, 1985.

Jolly, James. *The Classical Good CD and DVD Guide.* London: Gramophone, 2005.

The Kalevala: An Epic Poem after Oral Tradition by Elias Lönnrot. Translated by Keith Bosley. Oxford World's Classics. Oxford: Oxford University Press, 2009.

Kant, Immanuel. *Basic Writings of Kant.* Edited and with an introduction by Allen W. Wood. New York: Modern Library, 2001.

Kersten, Fred. *Galileo and the "Invention" of Opera: A Study in the Phenomenology of Consciousness.* Dordrecht, Netherlands: Kluwer Academic, 1997.

Kestenbaum, Victor. *The Grace and the Severity of the Ideal: John Dewey and the Transcendent.* Chicago: University of Chicago Press, 2002.

Klaver, Irene. "Silent Wolves." In *Wild Ideas*, 117–32. Edited by David Rothenberg. Minneapolis: University of Minnesota Press, 1995.

Krishnamurti, Jiddu. *Freedom from the Known.* San Francisco: Harper, 1969.

———. "Truth Is a Pathless Land." http://www.jkrishnamurti.org/about-krishnamurti/dissolution-speech.php

Kundera, Milan. *The Unbearable Lightness of Being.* Translated by Michael Henry Heim. New York: Harper & Row, 1984.

LeDoux, Joseph E. *The Emotional Brain: The Mysterious Underpinnings of Emotional Life.* New York: Simon & Schuster, 1996.

———. *Synaptic Self: How Our Brains Become Who We Are.* New York: Viking, 2001.

Levy-Bruhl, Lucien. *How Natives Think* [*Fonctions mentales dans les sociétés inférieures,* 1926]. Translated by Lilian A. Clare. Introductions by Lucien Levy-Bruhl and C. Scott Littleton. Princeton: Princeton University Press, 1985.

Lingis, Alphonso. *Excesses: Eros and Culture.* Albany: State University of New York Press, 1983.

Li Po. "The Ching-Ting Mountain." In *The Works of Li Po, the Chinese Poet, done into English verse by Shigeyoshi Obata,* 57. New York: Dutton, 1922.

Llinás, Rodolpho. *I of the Vortex: From Neurons to Self.* Cambridge, Mass.: The MIT Press, 2001.

Lowen, Alexander. *Bioenergetics.* New York: Penguin, 1975.

Lucretius. *Of the Nature of Things* [*De rerum natura*]. Translated by Thomas Creech [1682]. N.P.: Ulan Press, 2012.

Maggin, Donald L. *Stan Getz: A Life in Jazz.* New York: Harper Perennial, 1996.

Mahler, Gustav. Symphony no. 4. Pittsburgh Symphony Orchestra. André Previn. Angel Records SZ 537576, 1979, compact disc.

———. Symphony no. 4. City of Birmingham Symphony Orchestra. Simon Rattle. EMI 7243 5 56563, 1998, compact disc.

———. Symphony no. 6, *Tragic.* Cleveland Orchestra. George Szell. Sony Classical B000027OH, 1992, compact disc.

Marcel, Gabriel. *Gabriel Marcel's Perspectives on the Broken World: "The Broken World," a Four-Act Play, Followed by "Concrete Approaches to Investigating the Ontological Mystery."* Translated by Katharine R. Hanley. Milwaukee, Wis.: Marquette University Press, 1998.

———. *The Philosophy of Existentialism.* Translated by Manya Harari. New York: Carol Publishing, 1995.

Marshall, Robert. "The Problem of the Wilderness." *Scientific Monthly* 30, no. 2 (February 1930): 141–48.

Martin, Calvin Luther. *The Language of Wildness.* Work in progress, online access: http://yupik.wordpress.com

Masson, Jeffrey Moussaieff, and Susan McCarthy. *When Elephants Weep: The Emotional Lives of Animals.* New York: Delacorte, 1995.

McCullough, David. *John Adams.* New York: Simon & Schuster, 2001.

McManus, Jill. *Spring Is in the Air.* With Jill McManus (piano) and Bob Arkin (bass). Compact disc.

Midgley, Mary. *Beast and Man: The Roots of Human Nature.* Ithaca, N.Y.: Cornell University Press, 1978.

Miller, William Lee. *President Lincoln: The Duty of a Statesman*. New York: Knopf, 2008.

Minahan, John A. *Word Like a Bell: John Keats, Music and the Romantic Poet*. Kent, Oh.: Kent State University Press, 1992.

Morelle, Rebecca. "Dolphins 'Call Each Other by Name,'" BBC World Service, July 22, 2013, http://www.bbc.co.uk/news/science-environment-23410137.

Mozart, Wolfgang Amadeus. Symphonies nos. 32, 35, and 39. Prague Chamber Orchestra. Sir Charles Mackerras. Telarc, 2003, compact disc.

———. Symphonies nos. 40 and 41. Prague Chamber Orchestra. Sir Charles Mackerras. Telarc, 2003, compact disc.

Nabokov, Peter. *Native American Testimony: A Chronicle of Indian-White Relations from Prophecy to the Present, 1492–1992*. New York: Penguin, 1991.

Neihardt, John G. *Black Elk Speaks: Being the Life Story of a Holy Man of the Oglala Sioux*. 1932. Introduction by Vine Deloria Jr. Lincoln: University of Nebraska Press, 1979.

Nietzsche, Friedrich. *The Birth of Tragedy and The Case of Wagner*. Translated with commentary by Walter Kaufmann. New York: Vintage, 1967.

———. *The Gay Science*. Translated by Walter Kaufmann. New York: Vintage, 1974.

———. *Thus Spoke Zarathustra: A Book for All and None*. Translated by Walter Kaufmann. New York: Penguin, 1978.

———. *Twilight of the Idols and The Anti-Christ*. Translated by R. J. Hollingdale. Introduction by Michael Tanner. New York: Penguin, 1990.

———. *The Will to Power*. Edited and translated by Walter Kaufmann and R. J. Hollingdale. New York: Vintage, 1968.

Penrose, Roger. *The Emperor's New Mind: Concerning Computers, Minds and the Laws of Physics*. Oxford: Oxford University Press, 1989.

———. *Shadows of the Mind: A Search for the Missing Science of Consciousness*. Oxford: Oxford University Press, 1994.

Pert, Candace B., M.D. *The Molecules of Emotion: Why You Feel the Way You Feel*. Foreword by Deepak Chopra, M.D. New York: Scribner, 1997.

Petkova, Valeria I., and H. Henrik Ehrsson. "If I Were You: Perceptual Illusion of Body Swapping." www.PLoS ONE 3(12):e3832.doi:10.1371/journal.pone.0003832.

Peirce, Charles Sanders. *Collected Papers of Charles Sanders Peirce*. 8 vols. Cambridge, Mass.: Harvard University Press, 1931–58.

———. "The Law of Mind." *Monist* 2 (1891–92): 533–59. Reprinted in *Collected Papers of Charles Sanders Peirce*, 6:102–63.

Plato. *Apology*. In *The Trial and Death of Socrates: Four Dialogues*. Translated by Benjamin Jowett. New York: Classic Books International, 2010.

Pollan, Michael. *The Omnivore's Dilemma: A Natural History of Four Meals.* New York: Penguin, 2006.

Putnam, Ruth Anna, ed. *The Cambridge Companion to William James.* Cambridge: Cambridge University Press, 1997.

Rochberg, George. *The Aesthetics of Survival: A Composer's View of Twentieth-Century Music.* Edited and with an introduction by William Bolcom. Ann Arbor: University of Michigan Press, 1984.

———. Symphony No. 5 / *Black Sounds* / *Transcendental Variations.* Saarbrücken Radio Symphony. Christopher Lyndon-Gee. Naxos American Classics B00009L4W5, 2003, compact disc.

Sacks, Oliver. *Musicophilia: Tales of Music and the Brain.* Revised and expanded edition. New York: Vintage, 2008.

Sale, Kirkpatrick. *Human Scale.* New York: Coward, McCann & Geoghegen, 1980.

Sartre, Jean-Paul. *Being and Nothingness: An Essay on Phenomenological Ontology.* Translated by Hazel E. Barnes. New York: Philosophical Library, 1956.

———. *Sketch for a Theory of the Emotions.* 1939. Translated by Philip Mairet. New York: Routledge, 2003.

Schelling, F. W. J. *The Ages of the World.* Translated with an introduction by Jason M. Wirth. Albany: State University of New York Press, 2000.

Schnittke, Alfred. Symphony no. 2, *St Florian.* Russian State Symphony Orchestra. Valeri Polyansky. Liner notes by Alexander Ivashkin. Chandos 9519, 1997, compact disc.

Schoenberg, Arnold. *Verklärte Nacht*; Schubert, Franz. String Quintet in C Major. Hollywood String Quartet. Testament B000003XID, 1994, compact disc.

———. *The Romantic Music of Schoenberg: Verklärte Nacht, Pelleas und Melisande.* Atlanta Symphony. Telarc B000003D0B, 2002, compact disc.

Shorto, Russell. *The Island at the Center of the World: The Epic Story of Dutch Manhattan and the Forgotten Colony That Shaped America.* New York: Vintage, 2004.

Shostakovich, Dmitri. *Testimony: The Memoirs of Dmitri Shostakovich.* As related to and edited by Solomon Volkov. New York: Harper & Row, 1979.

Silko, Leslie Marmon. *Ceremony.* New York: Penguin, 1977.

Sloboda, John A. *The Musical Mind: The Cognitive Psychology of Music.* Oxford: Oxford University Press, 1986.

Some, Malidoma Patrice. *Of Water and the Spirit.* New York: Penguin, 1985.

Sophocles. *Oedipus, King of Thebes.* Translated by Gilbert Murray. London: George Allen & Unwin, 1911.

Suzuki, David, narrator and host. *The Sacred Balance*. Four-part documentary series directed and produced by Robert Lang. Kensington Communications. 2002.

———. *The Sacred Balance: Rediscovering Our Place in Nature*, Updated and Expanded. Vancouver, B.C., Canada: Greystone, 1997.

Thomas, Dylan. *A Child's Christmas in Wales*. Norfolk, Conn.: New Directions, 1954.

Thompson, Evan. "Neurophenomenology and Contemplative Experience." In *Oxford Handbook of Science and Religion*, 226–35. Edited by Philip Clayton and Zachary Simpson. Oxford: Oxford University Press, 2008.

Thoreau, Henry David. *Walden*. 1854. Introduction and annotations by Bill McKibben. Boston: Beacon, 1997.

———. "Walking." In *Henry David Thoreau: Collected Essays and Poems*. Edited by Elizabeth Hall Witherell. New York: Library of America, 2001.

Tiller, William. *Conscious Acts of Creation: The Emergence of a New Physics*. Walnut Creek, Calif.: Pavior, 2001.

———. *Psychoenergetic Science: A Second Copernican-Scale Revolution*. Walnut Creek, Calif.: Pavior, 2007.

———. *Science and Human Transformation: Subtle Energies, Intentionality and Consciousness*. Walnut Creek, Calif.: Pavior, 1997.

Tolstoy, Leo. *War and Peace: The Maude Translation, Backgrounds and Sources, Criticism*. Edited by George Gibion. Translated by Louise and Alymer Maude. New York: Norton, 1996.

Tversky, Amos, and Daniel Kahneman. "Judgment Under Uncertainty: Heuristics and Biases," *Science*, New Series, 185, no. 4157 (Sep. 27, 1974): 1124–31. Reprinted in *Judgment under Uncertainty: Heuristics and Biases*, ed. Daniel Kahneman, Paul Slovic, and Amos Tversky. Cambridge: Cambridge University Press, 1982.

Vidal, Gore. *Burr: A Novel*. New York: Random House, 1973.

Waters, Frank. *The Man Who Killed the Deer*. London: Neville Spearman, 1962.

Weil, Andrew, and Kimba Arem. *Self-Healing with Sound and Music*. Sounds True 1591791987, 2006, 2 compact discs.

Wilshire, Bruce W. *Get 'Em All! Kill 'Em!: Genocide, Terrorism, Righteous Communities*. Lanham, Md.: Lexington, 2006.

———. *The Primal Roots of American Philosophy: Pragmatism, Phenomenology, and Native American Thought*. University Park: Pennsylvania State University, 2000.

———. *Role Playing and Identity: The Limits of Theatre as Metaphor*. Bloomington: Indiana University Press, 1982.

———. *Wild Hunger: The Primal Roots of Modern Addiction*. Lanham, Md.: Rowman & Littlefield, 1998.

———. *William James and Phenomenology: A Study of "The Principles of Psychology."* Bloomington: Indiana University Press, 1968.

———, ed. *Romanticism and Evolution: The Nineteenth Century.* An anthology selected, edited, and with an introduction by Bruce Wilshire. New York: Capricorn, 1968.

———, ed. *William James: The Essential Writings.* Preface by James M. Edie. New York: Harper & Row, 1971.

Yeats, W. B. "Man and the Echo." In *The Collected Works of W. B. Yeats. Volume I: The Poems.* Revised Second Edition, 345. New York: Simon and Schuster, 2010.

———. "The Second Coming." In *The Collected Works of W. B. Yeats. Volume I: The Poems.* Revised Second Edition, 187. New York: Simon and Schuster, 2010.

Index

AMERICAN PHILOSOPHY

Douglas R. Anderson and Jude Jones, series editors

Kenneth Laine Ketner, ed., *Peirce and Contemporary Thought: Philosophical Inquiries.*

Max H. Fisch, ed., *Classic American Philosophers: Peirce, James, Royce, Santayana, Dewey, Whitehead, second edition.* Introduction by Nathan Houser.

John E. Smith, *Experience and God, second edition.*

Vincent G. Potter, *Peirce's Philosophical Perspectives.* Edited by Vincent Colapietro.

Richard E. Hart and Douglas R. Anderson, eds., *Philosophy in Experience: American Philosophy in Transition.*

Vincent G. Potter, *Charles S. Peirce: On Norms and Ideals, second edition.* Introduction by Stanley M. Harrison.

Vincent M. Colapietro, ed., *Reason, Experience, and God: John E. Smith in Dialogue.* Introduction by Merold Westphal.

Robert J. O'Connell, S.J., *William James on the Courage to Believe, second edition.*

Elizabeth M. Kraus, *The Metaphysics of Experience: A Companion to Whitehead's "Process and Reality," second edition.* Introduction by Robert C. Neville.

Kenneth Westphal, ed., *Pragmatism, Reason, and Norms: A Realistic Assessment—Essays in Critical Appreciation of Frederick L. Will.*

Beth J. Singer, *Pragmatism, Rights, and Democracy.*

Eugene Fontinell, *Self, God, and Immorality: A Jamesian Investigation.*

Roger Ward, *Conversion in American Philosophy: Exploring the Practice of Transformation.*

Michael Epperson, *Quantum Mechanics and the Philosophy of Alfred North Whitehead.*

Kory Sorrell, *Representative Practices: Peirce, Pragmatism, and Feminist Epistemology.*

Naoko Saito, *The Gleam of Light: Moral Perfectionism and Education in Dewey and Emerson.*

Josiah Royce, *The Basic Writings of Josiah Royce.*

Douglas R. Anderson, *Philosophy Americana: Making Philosophy at Home in American Culture.*

James Campbell and Richard E. Hart, eds., *Experience as Philosophy: On the World of John J. McDermott.*

John J. McDermott, *The Drama of Possibility: Experience as Philosophy of Culture.* Edited by Douglas R. Anderson.

Larry A. Hickman, *Pragmatism as Post-Postmodernism: Lessons from John Dewey.*

Larry A. Hickman, Stefan Neubert, and Kersten Reich, eds., *John Dewey Between Pragmatism and Constructivism.*

Dwayne A. Tunstall, *Yes, But Not Quite: Encountering Josiah Royce's Ethico-Religious Insight.*

Josiah Royce, *Race Questions, Provincialism, and Other American Problems, ex̣panded edition*. Edited by Scott L. Pratt and Shannon Sullivan.

Lara Trout, *The Politics of Survival: Peirce, Affectivity, and Social Criticism.*

John R. Shook and James A. Good, *John Dewey's Philosophy of Spirit, with the ǻšôẩ Lecture on Hegel.*

Josiah Warren, *The Practical Anarchist: Writings of Josiah Warren*. Edited and with an Introduction by Crispin Sartwell.

Naoko Saito and Paul Standish, eds., *Stanley Cavell and the Education of Grownups.*

Douglas R. Anderson and Carl R. Hausman, *Conversations on Peirce: Reals and Ideals.*

Rick Anthony Furtak, Jonathan Ellsworth, and James D. Reid, eds., *Thoreau's Importance for Philosophy.*

James M. Albrecht, *Reconstructing Individualism: A Pragmatic Tradition from Emerson to Ellison.*

Mathew A. Foust, *Loyalty to Loyalty: Josiah Royce and the Genuine Moral Life.*

Cornelis de Waal and Krysztof Piotr Skowroński (eds.), *The Normative Thought of Charles S. Peirce.*

Dwayne A. Tunstall, *Doing Philosophy Personally: Thinking about Metaphysics, Theism, and Antiblack Racism.*

Erin McKenna, *Pets, People, and Pragmatism.*

Sami Pihlström, *Pragmatic Pluralism and the Problem of God.*

Thomas Alexander, *The Human Eros: Eco-ontology and the Aesthetics of Ex̣istence.*

John Kaag, *Thinking Through the Imagination: Aesthetics in Human Cognition.*

Kelly A. Parker and Jason Bell (eds.), *The Relevance of Royce.*

W. E. B. Du Bois, *The Problem of the Color Line at the Turn of the Twentieth Century: The Essential Early Essays*. Edited by Nahum Dimitri Chandler.

Nahum Dimitri Chandler, *X—The Problem of the Negro as a Problem for Thought.*

John Lachs, *Freedom and Limits*. Edited by Patrick Shade.

Morris Grossman, *Art and Morality: Essays in the Spirit of George Santayana*. Edited by Martin A. Coleman.

Peter Hare, *Pragmatism with Purpose: Selected Writings*. Edited by Joseph Palencik, Douglas R. Anderson, and Steven A. Miller.

Hermann Deuser, Hans Joas, Matthias Jung, and Magnus Schlette (eds.), *The Varieties of Transcendence: Pragmatism and the Theory of Religion.*

Bruce W. Wilshire, *The Much-at-Once: Music, Science, Ecstasy, the Body*. Foreword by Edward S. Casey.